Dr. Earl Mindell's

What You Should Know About Herbs for Your Health

Dr. Earl Mindell's

What You Should Know About Herbs for Your Health

Earl L. Mindell, R.Ph., Ph.D.

with Virginia L. Hopkins

Keats Publishing, Inc.　　New Canaan, Connecticut

DR. EARL MINDELL'S WHAT YOU SHOULD KNOW ABOUT HERBS FOR YOUR HEALTH

Copyright © 1996 by Earl L. Mindell

All Rights Reserved

No part of this book may be reproduced in any form without the written consent of the publisher.

Library of Congress Cataloging-in-Publication Data is available.

ISBN 0-87983-749-7

Printed in the United States of America

Keats Publishing, Inc.
27 Pine Street (Box 876)
New Canaan, Connecticut 06840-0876

99 98 97 96   6 5 4 3 2 1

CONTENTS

ACKNOWLEDGMENTS

We would like to thank Maria Gordon, Larry Johns and Kim Shepherd for their invaluable assistance in writing this book.

PART I
Herbs, Folklore and Pharmacy

Herbs, the Original Medicines

Can you imagine a world without bottles of aspirin and antibiotics? How would you feel if your doctor had no drugs to prescribe for serious illnesses? This was the world of our not-so-distant ancestors and, what's more, it still exists today in Third World countries. Yet it is precisely this primitive world that we owe for all the benefits of modern medicine we enjoy.

The pharmaceutical industry has learned to harness the power of many natural substances, producing synthetic versions which have become our prescription and over-the-counter drugs. These have brought undoubted advances, but often at the cost of debilitating side effects and complications.

Meanwhile, more and more scientific research is serving to remind us of nature's own safer, gentler packages of healing power which lie behind so many of today's drugs. The truth is that remedies like Grandma's elderberry wine and the Chickasaw Indians' infusion of willow root are scientifically proven! As more and more natural remedies are tested and refined, the apparent need for expensive drugs with dangerous side effects declines. Science is showing real medical advances are in store as we learn to combine old wisdom with new.

WHAT IS AN HERB?

Any plant with medicinal properties is called an herb. Of course, herbs can also be plants used as food, or in cosmetics, or for seasoning or flavoring. Herbs used to treat physical conditions are plants that in some way demonstrate a healing effect.

Herbs are the main source of medicine for the primary care needs of possibly 80 percent of the world's population. This was the World Health Organization's estimate in 1985. In the U.S. herbs have been overtaken by manufactured drugs only in the past 60 years. Until World War II, the *U.S. Pharmacopoeia*, the listing of officially accepted medicines, included herbal preparations. Even today, nearly 40 percent of prescribed drugs dispensed in the U.S. are either based on or are synthesized versions of natural substances. In a way, herbs could be said to be the forgotten or hidden healing element of modern medicine.

CHAPTER 1

The Ancient Tradition of Herbal Medicines

Chrysanthemum as an antibiotic? It's true, and, would you believe it, used by chimpanzees! Zoologists in Africa have seen one species regularly dosing themselves with this potent plant. All of us have seen sick cats and dogs eating grass. Imagine human intelligence and curiosity combined with instinct, and it's easy to see how prehistoric cultures must have developed considerable knowledge of the medicinal properties of the plants around them.

We no longer have to chew on buckthorn and discover its purgative effects by accident! Someone long ago ate lobelia flowers and ended up with their head over an ancient toilet. It is modern science that labels these things as laxatives and emetics, but it was wise, observant people of the past who discovered them and realized that their actions could relieve illness. Indeed, the remains of plants known as herbal remedies such as bramble, crab apple, orache (a spinach-like weed) and wild service tree have been found in the pots and waste pits of Neolithic villages in England and Switzerland. The recording of such remedies began as civilization advanced, allowing us to trace fascinating herbal treatments from every culture far back into history.

Traditional herbal medicine in India, called Ayurveda, goes back more than 5,000 years. As far back as 3,000 B.C., official schools of herbalism existed in Egypt, teaching about plants like garlic, mint, and coriander. Cleopatra is said to have used cucumber to preserve her skin and the *Ebers Papryus*, written about 1,500 B.C., recommends applying a moldy piece of bread to open wounds, thousands of years before Alexander Fleming developed penicillin from the very same mold.

The Chinese were using oil from hydnocarpus trees to treat leprosy as early as 2,500 B.C. Centuries later came the *Shen Nong Ben Cao Jing*, China's first true herbal, describing more than 350 plants used for medicinal purposes. The Chinese were also using ephedrine, our over-the-counter cold medication, in the form of the shrub ma huang, over two thousand years ago.

Although a religious work, the Bible is another rich source of herbal references from cinnamon to myrrh, with mandrakes even serving as aphrodisiacs in the Genesis story of Jacob's wives, Leah and Rachel.

Early European settlers in America were amazed at and often thankful for the range of medicinal applications for herbs used by the Indians for needs from headaches to heart conditions. Tribes such as the Iroquois and Mohegans treated colds and fevers with tea made from the boneset plant. Wormwood was a bronchitis and cold remedy used by Indians as far apart as New Mexico and British Columbia. Thompson Indians would stuff their nostrils with wormwood leaves to relieve nasal congestion and when burying decaying corpses! As America was settled, remedies were exchanged. Europeans for example learned of soothing witch hazel ointment from the North Americans, and Indians learned to use dandelion remedies for conditions like heartburn as the plant was introduced to their country.

Some American Indian, and European, and Eastern remedies were often selected in a similar manner, referred to as the Doctrine of Signatures. A plant would be used to treat a condition of a body part which it resembled. Liverleaf, with liver-shaped leaves, for example, was used to treat liver disorders. Science has even proven links for plants such as red bloodroot as a "blood purifier" and the yellowish goldenseal root for the treatment of jaundice.

European herbal remedies, passed down through village wise women, sold by wandering herbalists, and often copied by monks from ancient Greek and Roman writings, were used by royalty and peasants alike. Queen Elizabeth I is said to have favored meadowsweet, used to treat flu, fever and arthritis. From Roman times, lavender was known to promote relaxation, while chervil was recommended as a stimulant—one that also reportedly cured hiccups if you ate the whole plant! Arabs, too, used Greek and Roman texts, elaborating on remedies with often highly sweetened preparations and exotic spices. Herbs such as ginger and cardamom were believed to prevent illness.

The herbals of 16th and 17th century Europe make colorful reading today. Would you swallow sumac powder if you were advised that it had "great efficacy in strengthening the stomach and bowels?" Would you wash "pestiferous sores" with wild succory? How about calamint to kill "all manner of worms in the body"? We might smile and raise our eyebrows at some of these ancient herbal treatments, but science today is telling us loud and clear that many a plant prescription makes as much, if not more sense, than a modern drug equivalent.

CHAPTER 2

From Folklore to Pharmaceutical

Observation, trial and error, and faith seem to have been key to the practice of early Western herbalism. It came with no real system or rules until the second century A.D. and a Greek called Galen, physician to a Roman Emperor. Galen's Herbal marked the beginning of a trend separating the professional physician from the traditional healer. Influenced by Galen and his rigid rules, medicine began to be taught in Europe as a superior art favoring exotic medicines with aggressive treatments such as bloodletting and purging.

Following the failure of this style of doctoring to help in the Black Plague of 1348 and again with outbreaks of syphilis, Galenic practice began to be challenged in Europe in the 16th and 17th centuries. Herbalists such as the famous Englishman, Nicholas Culpeper, helped expose the false mystery and monopoly of "official" medicine and brought simple, garden-grown remedies back to popularity. Brutal attempts at dramatic cures with practices like medical bleeding eventually died out, but not before George Washington was bled to death in 1797 during treatment for a sore throat.

The Swiss physician and alchemist, Paracelsus, who developed laudanum, also influenced the return to the idea that medicines were found by searching for cures held by plants. He even predicted that pharmacologically "active principles" would be found in

7

herbs. Ironically, it may have been the observation of just such active compounds in the plant, digitalis, that set orthodox medicine on the path of the synthetic drugs that came to replace herbs. In 1785, the English doctor William Withering detailed the biological effects and recommended doses of the plant digitalis. His work led eventually to the discovery of the modern heart stimulants digoxin and digitoxin.

Digitalis probably helped standard physicians continue to focus on the idea of the quick fix, in demand, too, of course, by the public. Although figures like Thomas Jefferson still cultivated herbs in kitchen gardens, 18th century chemists worked hard in laboratories to isolate and synthesize active ingredients and bypass the plants themselves. In this way, the modern pharmaceutical industry was born.

In a move to help companies recover the costs of research and development of synthetic substances, the American government passed a patent medicine law in the late 1800s. This gave companies the exclusive 17-year rights to sell patented drugs. Unfortunately, it also gave them an incentive to discredit the use of natural remedies in order to maximize profits from synthetic ones. Formation of the Federal Drug Administration (FDA) made the situation even worse for natural remedies. There is no incentive at all to gain FDA approval for an herbal medicine when it takes 10 to 18 years and costs millions of dollars with no patent protection at the end of it all!

In countries like France and Germany, however, the system for approval of medicines is different, and many natural medications are sold over-the-counter and prescribed. No health claims can be made in America for herbal remedies, which must be sold as foods or supplements. Thanks also to the American Medical Association (AMA) support and huge marketing campaigns, it's not surprising that synthetic drugs have dominated American medical teaching and treatment since the 1950s. However, surveys show the majority of Americans take supplements of some sort, and increasing numbers of physicians are beginning to integrate modern and traditional practices. The Program in Integrative Medicine at the University of Arizona, for example, is part of a new teaching trend which integrates alternative medicine with mainstream medicine. The future could take a very different path.

CHAPTER 3

Natural or Synthetic? A Question of Balance

Heart attack? Broken leg? Life-threatening infection? Western emergency treatment is the proven choice. But it's estimated that emergencies make up only about 20 percent of conditions treated by doctors. Viral infections, degenerative diseases, cancers, auto-immune diseases and other illnesses make up the other 80 percent. With the majority of illnesses, the focus of modern medicine has been the relief of symptoms. The aim with herbal remedies, on the other hand, is the restoration of health by treating the underlying cause.

Early herbalists regarded themselves as "nature's servants" and respected the body's natural efforts to return to wellness. Western pharmaceutical companies act more like nature's masters, attempting to manipulate biochemical functions in isolation from each other. The drugs they produce are concentrated versions of compounds recognized by the cells of our bodies. This is why they achieve their often fast and dramatic effects. However, to make an effective substance patentable, drug companies must add molecules that make the drug synthetic, or not found in nature. These extra molecules create additional biological reactions as they are processed—reactions we call side effects.

In contrast, herbal remedies package their active chemicals with beneficial substances that ameliorate side effects. This packaging can make the active compound more easily absorbed, as with the uptake of iron aided by the vitamin C in plants like watercress and rose hips. Other chemical combinations in herbs seem to be built-in safety measures. Ephedrine, isolated from the ma huang plant, was once prescribed for asthma, but produced the side effect of dangerously high blood pressure levels. The whole plant has been used for thousands of years with no harmful results. The difference? Six related chemicals in the herb itself, one of which actually lowers blood pressure and reduces heart rate. Aspirin can relieve pain and fever, but may cause stomach bleeding. Its natural derivative, white willow bark, is without this unwanted effect.

Scientific analysis bears out the observation that the effects of chemicals in plants often have parallel effects in humans. Plants such as cranberries contain substances which help to preserve them by killing bacteria. The same substances have similar effects in our bodies. This sort of phenomenon is not surprising, as every living thing is made of the same basic constituents such as proteins and sugars, and since they have all evolved from the same origins.

Medicinal plants also echo the body's own life-maintaining system of checks and balances. Ginseng, for instance, contains hormone-like substances called saponins. Some have a sedative effect, others are stimulating. The body, then, will naturally utilize the different saponins according to its needs. Ginseng, as a result, is a body stabilizer, increasing the ability of the body to withstand stress. Hawthorn berries work on blood pressure in the same way with a mixture of compounds which either raise or lower blood pressure. Expert herbalists are able to extend this process by creating remedies which are a combination of plants with a selected balance of effects.

Western medicine's pill-popping habits have led to passive, often fearful, but unquestioning patients who do not expect to take much part in their own recovery. Herbal medicine differs in that it demands a review of the body's overall condition as well as specific symptoms. Herbs themselves, and the way they are used, are more likely than synthetic drugs to address underlying conditions. The care, cultivation and mixing of herbs also brings respect for and conservation of natural resources.

While the advances brought about by modern medicine are obvious, Western levels of conditions like heart disease, hypertension and cancer are appallingly high. Complications from prescription drugs result in 40 percent of hospitalizations and cause 20,000 to 30,000 deaths every year in the United States. Yet, this is an age where a balance can be struck. Powerful, short-term treatment with synthetic drugs is a proven option. Gentle, safe, longer-term herbal medications deserve a role alongside as nature's complete pharmacy, evolved in natural harmony with the human body.

SCIENCE PROVES THE VALUE OF HERBS

Slaves building the Egyptian pyramids once went on strike over their rations of garlic! Today they would have scientific proof of its benefits—so much of it that even the U.S. medical establishment cannot falsely claim that none exists. Recent years have produced 2,000 studies on garlic by researchers all over the world. It has been shown to be antimicrobial, antibiotic, antiviral, antiparasitic, anticancer and an immune booster. Substances found in garlic include antioxidants, smooth muscle relaxants and four powerful anti-clotting agents. Studies have shown how these substances help garlic prevent and relieve heart disease. Garlic also inhibits an enzyme which generates an inflammatory chemical, explaining claims for its use with asthma.

Another ancient remedy proven effective by science is chamomile, used for centuries in Europe against infections and aches. Modern analysis shows it is an antispasmodic in the bowel and stomach with a sedative effect on the central nervous system. It also contains anti-inflammatories which contribute to its usefulness in ointments and lotions.

A North American remedy now validated scientifically is the purple coneflower, echinacea. This plant was used medicinally by native Indians more than any other plant. Echinacea treatments existed for wounds, burns, abscesses, insect bites, snake bites, toothache, joint pains and infections. Chemical analysis of echinacea reveals a fascinating combination of substances, including some with antiviral and anticancer properties and others which regenerate tissue. Interestingly, the antibiotic properties of echinacea are mild. Instead, scientists have found it is the strong immune enhancing activity of echinacea compounds which lie behind its power against internal and external bacterial infections.

A popular folk remedy for colds and flu, elderberry, has high concentrations of bioflavonoids. These could account for the recently proven ability of elderberry extract to kill flu viruses. A recent double-blind study using the commercial elderberry extract Sambucol more than halved the recovery time for sufferers of flu compared to subjects given placebos. As a winter tonic, elderberry is now official.

Chemicals called PCOs are the main effective agents in another berry, the bilberry or European blueberry. Bilberry jam was eaten to improve the night vision of

World War II pilots. Bilberry extract has indeed been shown to improve the ability of the eyes to adapt from dark to light. It also prevents and retard cataracts and ulcers and lowers blood sugar, so proving its folk use in the treatment of diagnosis. What's more, its smooth muscle relaxing effects have been demonstrated in experiments, showing exactly why it became a treatment for vascular disorders.

Another excellent example of an herb which shines under the spotlight of modern science is ginger. Used for thousands of years in China, ginger is shown to be high in antioxidants, to inhibit inflammation triggers and blood clotting agents, to kill bacteria and reduce cholesterol levels. Animal studies confirm ginger's historic use in warming the body and treating ulcers.

Experiments also show important differences in the composition of dry and raw ginger. They serve, too, to show why the effects of herbs like garlic and licorice change depending on their form. The standards of modern analysis and testing producing these kinds of observations give added reassurance to users of herbal remedies. They form a technological supplement to the huge volume of historical evidence for the efficacy of herbs. And they often stem, ironically, from the research used to produce synthetic drugs! Perhaps the pendulum is due now to rest between traditional herbal and modern medicines.

THE RACE FOR MODERN HERBAL DISCOVERIES IS ON

Did you know a major ingredient of birth control pills comes from wild yam or that quinine, the malaria drug, is derived from the Peruvian "fever tree," the cinchona? A surprising amount of the world's harvest goes to help produce the drugs of our time. Unhappily, the potential harvest has been dwindling at an amazing rate as land is cleared or developed. Experts like Tom Eisner, Schurman Professor of Biology at Cornell, point out that only about 2 percent of known plant species have been analyzed thoroughly for their pharmacological effects. Even worse, botanists estimate that millions of plants have still to be named and many have already been lost forever to environmental destruction. Only recently, logging operations in Pacific northwest forests burned Pacific yew as slash. Then came the discovery of the anti-cancer drug, taxol, in, yes, the bark of the Pacific yew tree. There is no doubt that many effective compounds must have already been lost as unknown species have been wiped out.

Naturalists and scientists have been spurred to work together to fully investigate the wealth of species already collected and to campaign for environmental preservation measures. The profit motive actually brings the cooperation of drug companies, too, which continually search for new plant drugs to synthesize. The payoff can be big, in medical and money terms, with finds like the rosy periwinkle, which has produced two anticancer drugs used successfully to treat childhood leukemias and Hodgkin's disease. This was an accidental spin-off of a drug company's search for antidiabetic agents. Drugs like the fungus-derived cyclosporin, an immune suppressant used in organ transplants, and ivermectin, a parasitic worm killer, have also been uncovered relatively recently.

Only a small percentage of known plants has already yielded tremendous medical benefit. It's simply common sense to continue the research and investigation of the depleted stocks of laboratory Earth while ensuring, too, that we don't burn down the laboratory itself.

MEDICINAL HERBS IN OTHER CULTURES

Because herbs are the main form of medicine for most cultures of the world, and pharmaceutical drugs are, relatively speaking, much more expensive and cause thousands of deaths every year, the World Health Organization is studying and promoting herbal medicines. Natural medicines have come into their own as inexpensive, safe and effective treatments easily accessible to their native users. There is a real opportunity for developing cultures to integrate natural remedies with the benefits of modern medicine and none of the penalties.

China, with its established and ancient herbal tradition, has been integrating positive aspects of Western medicine faster than natural remedies have been revived in the West. A revival is happening, however, and on an international scale. Many physicians from India also train in the U.S. and Europe, blending Ayurvedic and Western medicine in their practices. Scientific research has spurred fresh interest, seeing sales of herbal products pass $4 billion in Germany alone, and higher figures in Japan.

Use of herbal remedies as standard medicines in different countries probably never dipped as low as they did in the U.S. with its restrictive FDA regulations. Herbal medicines and modern drugs face the same legal tests in Germany, and insurance reimburses the costs of herbal remedies sold in pharmacies when they are prescribed by a doctor. One of the top three most widely prescribed drugs in both Germany and France is ginkgo biloba, used to treat certain vascular disorders. In the U.S., gingko biloba can only be sold as a food supplement. German physicians might also prescribe the herb valerian to treat mild anxiety. Homeopathic remedies are very widely prescribed in France. In Great Britain, natural remedies have always sat side by side with synthetic remedies on drug store shelves.

Around the world, cultural gravity seems to be working to pull Western medicine back down to its herbal roots. The weight of scientific evidence only adds to the pull, with the message that stronger links with nature are good medicine everywhere on Earth.

PART II
A Guide to My Favorite Healing Herbs

CHAPTER 4

How to Use the Healing Herbs

As modern technology becomes increasingly sophisticated, we are discovering more and more about just how complex plant ingredients are. We used to believe that beta-carotene was the only useful vitamin in a carrot. Now we know that in a raw carrot there are hundreds of carotenoids, of which beta-carotene is only one. In addition, a raw carrot is packed with vitamins, minerals, sugars, enzymes, fibers, and dozens of other substances we don't fully understand yet.

Think of celery and lettuce. For years we were told they had no nutritional value. Now we know that if you eat six stalks of celery a day your blood pressure will almost certainly drop. Lettuce contains ingredients that can make you sleepy. It's not that these vegetables had no nutritional value, it's just that until recently, our technology and science weren't advanced enough to understand them!

Any healing herb or medicinal plant is a veritable chemistry lab of ingredients with specific biochemical actions and reactions in the human body. These include volatile oils which give plants their aroma, sterols which have similarities to our own steroid hormones, saponins which have "soapy" qualities, and alkaloids, which are often poisonous to the liver but which sometimes have profound healing properties.

Each healing herb listed here has specific effects on the body, based on its chemical makeup. The chemicals that have the strongest effects on the tissues and organs of the body are called *active principles*. Plants rich in active principles are the most valuable as medicines. It is the active principles in plants that the pharmaceutical companies attempt to isolate, patent and turn into pharmaceutical drugs. But what we have found, over and over again, is that once an active principle is isolated from the other ingredients in a plant, it has side effects. Somehow in the miraculous wisdom of nature, a whole herb prepared and taken properly has very few if any, side effects. The synergy or combination of ingredients working together in a plant brings a balance to it as a medicine that makes herbal medicine gentle and yet still effective.

While herbal medicines are more gentle than pharmaceutical drugs, don't be fooled into thinking that herbs can be used carelessly. A wide range of potency and toxicity exists among the healing herbs. Women who are pregnant or nursing, and anyone with a serious chronic illness such as diabetes or heart disease, should carefully research an herb, or consult with a health care professional familiar with herbs, before using it.

For example, angelica can be a wonderful herb for indigestion, and for inducing sweating in a cold. But because it increases circulation, it can also promote menstruation, so it shouldn't be used by pregnant women. Another active principle in angelica can cause it to increase the amount of sugar in the blood, so it shouldn't be used by diabetics without supervision.

Your doctor is unlikely to encourage you to use herbal medicine. He or she was told in medical school that herbs were unscientific, superstitious folklore. Doctors are trained that their job is to diagnose a disease and then find a drug to prescribe for the symptoms of the disease. While I know that you're going to get a negative response ranging from condescension to dire warnings if you tell your doctor you're taking herbs, I encourage you not to self-treat yourself with herbs if you have a serious or chronic condition. Seek out a doctor who uses natural medicines, or find a naturopathic doctor. Many chiropractors are also skilled in the use of natural medicines.

IF YOU'RE TAKING OTHER MEDICATIONS

I want you to be aware that mixing herbs with pharmaceutical drugs can cause the drug to overreact or underreact. For example, ephedra may help dry up your sinuses, but it also can raise blood pressure and increase heart rate, which could be dangerous for someone taking a heart drug. In another example, echinacea won't interfere with an antibiotic, but because it stimulates the immune system, it could interfere with an immunosuppressive drug such as a cortisone.

On the other side of the coin, taking herbs that support your body can help alleviate the side effects of a prescription drug. For example, if you're taking acetaminophen (Tylenol), which is very hard on the liver, taking milk thistle (silymarin) will help support your liver.

I realize you can't possibly figure out all the possible interactions of drugs, foods and herbs, but I want you to be aware that herbs do have specific biochemical actions in the body and use caution. My best advice to you is to use common sense and moderation, and follow the proper dosage instructions.

As a pharmacist I am well aware that no two people respond to a medicine in the same way. Each person's biochemistry is unique. Your weight, age, sex, how much you exercise, your diet, and whether you use drugs such as alcohol and caffeine, will all affect how you respond to an herbal medicine.

If you try an herb and feel worse, stop taking it. If you try an herb and nothing happens, try half again to twice as much. If there is still no result, this probably isn't the herb for you. (Some herbs take 2-4 weeks to affect the system in a noticeable way. Again, do your research.)

IF YOU'RE PREGNANT

When you're pregnant you want to avoid putting anything in your body that would disrupt or interfere with the growth of the fetus. Please don't take herbs of any kind if you're pregnant without checking first with an experienced health professional familiar with herbs. There are a few herbs, such as raspberry leaf, which can be beneficial to take when you're pregnant, and there are specific herbs to help with labor and to start breast milk flowing. However, these should only be used with an experienced professional.

DO YOUR RESEARCH

Before taking any herb, do your homework. That could be as simple as referring to this book, or it could mean buying a more detailed herb book and doing some in-depth research. Don't use an herb long-term without thoroughly checking it out. Powerful herbs such as ephedra should never be used for more than a week or two at a time.

CHAPTER 5

My Top Twenty-Nine Healing Herbs

ARNICA (Arnica montana)

Also commonly called leopard's bane, arnica is a perennial herb found singly or in small clusters in mountainous regions. Its bright yellow, daisy-like flower heads bloom around July.

The volatile oils from the dried flower heads of European arnica have been used since the 11th century largely as a topical pain reliever and as an application to treat bruises and sprains. The Catawba Indians used a tea of arnica root resins for treating back pains. In old Russia, the herb was used internally to reduce cholesterol, promote production of bile, stimulate the nervous system, stop bleeding and to strengthen the heart.

Externally, the classic use of arnica is for muscle, joint or cartilage pain which is generally aggravated by movement and alleviated by rest. Typically, arnica is rubbed on the skin to soothe and heal bruises, sprains, hyperextensions, wounds, irritations and to provide relief due to muscle spasm, arthritis or bursitis. Placed on the stomach, a compress containing arnica can relieve abdominal pains. Applied as a salve, arnica is also good for chapped lips, irritated nostrils and acne. Only a highly diluted form of arnica should be used when the surface of the skin is broken. Too strong a concentration can cause blistering. There are a wide variety of arnica creams and salves available at your health food store.

Internally, tinctures of arnica are used for mental and physical shock, pain and swelling, concussion, fractured bones, sprains, dental extractions and headache. Some doctors have used the herb for internal bleeding, obstinate sore throat and inflammation of the mouth. Arnica should never be used internally without medical direction because an overdose can be fatal.

Arnica works by stimulating activity of white blood cells (macrophages) that perform much of the digestion of congested blood and by dispersing trapped, disorganized fluids from banged, bumped and bruised tissues, muscles and joints.

ALOE VERA (Aloe barbadensis)

It's common to see a spiky house plant with thick, rubbery, tapering green leaves edged with spiny teeth in a pot sitting around homes. Those wise to the ways of herbal healing keep it in the kitchen. The plant is aloe vera, or lily of the desert, and for most people it is there waiting to exude a mucilaginous sap when broken as first aid to quickly spread over a burn to relieve pain and prevent blisters. However, the skin-healing properties of aloe are not limited to burns.

In Africa, prior to hunting, natives rub the gel of the aloe over their bodies to remove the human scent. Women all over the world apply aloe gel on their skin to keep it supple and to clear blemishes. Greek history records the use of aloe as a healing herb for wounds 2,000 years ago. Legend has it Cleopatra massaged the gel into her skin every day. Napoleon's wife, Josephine, is said to have used a lotion of aloe and milk for her complexion.

In Ayurvedic medicine, aloe gel is a tonic for the female reproductive system. At one time people rubbed it into their scalps, believing it prevented hair loss. The gel is used to treat ulcers, ring worms, shingles, and to repel insects.

Aloe reportedly helps to clear pimples and acne. Dermatologists have also had success treating oily skin, dandruff, and psoriasis. By applying aloe to their nipples, nursing mothers can begin to reduce the supply of milk, thereby serving as an aid to weaning. And, aloe has been found to aid in the treatment of frostbite.

The medicinal properties of aloe have now been scientifically substantiated. Research documents its healing effect of all kinds of burns and the itch caused by poison ivy and oak. Additional studies have confirmed the anesthetic, antibacterial, and tissue restorative properties of this remarkable herb. The gel does indeed heal burns from the sun or a hot pan, and when not severe, regenerates tissue without scarring.

Aloe is believed to improve wound healing by increasing the availability of oxygen and by increasing the synthesis and strength of collagen and tissue.

BILBERRY (Vaccinium myrtillus)

The bilberry, or European blueberry, is a perennial shrub that grows in meadows and woods in Europe. Only the blue-black berries of the plant are used. These differ from the American blueberry in that the meat of the bilberry fruit is blue-black throughout.

Bilberry has long been a folk remedy for poor vision and "night blindness." During World War II, British Royal Air Force pilots reported improved vision on night bombing raids after eating bilberry jam.

Clinical tests confirm that bilberry given orally to humans not only improves visual accuracy in healthy people, but also helps those with eye diseases such as pigmentosa, retinitis, glaucoma and myopia. Components in the herb work specifically to improve vision by improving microcirculation and speeding the regeneration of retinal purple, a substance required for good eyesight.

Bilberry extract has been widely used in connection with vascular, or blood vessel disorders. Specific studies reveal a positive effect in the treatment of varicose veins, thrombosis and angina. The active components of bilberries are its flavonoids, which serve to prevent capillary fragility, inhibit platelet aggregation and stimulate the release of vasodilators, substances which open up blood vessels and improve the flow of blood, thus increasing the level of oxygen in tissues.

Recent research has also indicated that bilberry extract possesses significant preventive and curative anti-ulcer properties, attributed to the strengthening of the defensive barriers of the digestive system.

CALENDULA (Calendula officinalis)

A featured plant in many ornamental gardens, calendula or pot marigold, is a hardy, many-branched annual, almost entirely covered with fine hairs. The yellow-to-deep orange flowers ray out from a central head and close up at night.

Ancient Romans named this plant, noting that the flowers were in bloom on the first day, or calends, of every month. They also grew calendulas to treat scorpion bites. In early use, the herb was also used to treat headaches, fevers and toothaches. A 16th century concoction which called for the use of calendula was thought to enable one to see fairies.

Calendula came to America with settlers from Europe and was used during the Civil War to help stop bleeding and promote the healing of wounds.

Medically, calendula flower tinctures have been recommended in the treatment of a wide variety of ailments, including fever, cramps, flu, and stomach aches. Others apply calendula-based remedies to external sores, cuts, bruises, burns and rashes. Calendula flowers are said to relieve the pain of bee stings. And when applied directly to the ear, calendula oil can reduce earache pain. Mothers find it works well as a solution for diaper rash. Calendula and arnica are often combined in commercial skin ointments for burns and bruises.

Calendula tea can be used as an eye wash for sore, reddened eyes. As a cosmetic, calendula brings out highlights in blond and brunette hair, and is found in herbal bath mixtures to stimulate the body.

The flavor and color of calendula account for its widespread use in cooking, particularly soups, cheeses and salads.

The volatile oils in calendula stimulate blood circulation and induce sweating, thus aiding fevers to break, and accelerate eruptions like measles or rashes. Calendula also increases urinating, aids digestion and acts as a general tonic. The herb's antiseptic value is likely related to its content of natural iodine.

CAT'S CLAW (Uncaria tomentosa)

We keep hearing about the medical potential of plants growing undiscovered in the Amazon jungles of South America. One that is showing great potential as an healing herb has been brought to this country. It is called cat's claw, or una de gato, its Spanish name.

Scientific studies on cat's claw are in progress, but Indians native to the Amazon rain forest have long relied on this herb to heal a range of ills. Although many, many claims have been made for the various healing powers of cat's claw, studies on it are limited.

The herb does, however, seem to hold promise for enhancing the immune system and as an anti-inflammatory, meaning it may well deliver relief from joint pain, like arthritis.

At this time, scientists have not isolated the active constituents of cat's claw in their quest to manufacture a patentable drug. In other words, the whole plant works very effectively, but there doesn't seem to be one single ingredient that's responsible for its healing powers.

If you have arthritis, you may want to try cat's claw, particularly if other things you have tried for inflammatory conditions have proved unsuccessful.

One caution: natives of Peru reportedly use cat's claw for birth control, so please don't take it if you are attempting to become pregnant.

DONG QUAI (Angelica sinensis)

This fragrant perennial herb grows in China, Korea, and Japan. The root of the plant is described as having a head, body and tail to correspond with the herb's various applications.

The reputation of dong quai in Asia is second only to ginseng. Regarded as the ultimate, all-purpose woman's tonic herb, it is used for almost every gynecological complaint, from regulating the menstrual cycle and treating menopausal symptoms, such as hot flashes caused by hormonal changes, to assuring a healthy pregnancy and easy delivery. Chinese women have used dong quai for centuries to stop painful menstrual cramps caused by uterine contractions.

Herbalists today use dong quai for menopausal symptoms such as hot flashes, PMS, and to stimulate regular menstruation when women go off birth control pills.

Scientific investigation has shown that dong quai

produces a balancing effect on estrogen activity. The herb, rich in vitamins and minerals, has also been used to promote blood circulation and correct anemia in both sexes, as well as to treat insomnia, lower high blood pressure, and to alleviate constipation.

Most recently, studies involving dong quai have indicated that the herb regulates irregular heart beat, may help prevent heart disease, and acts as an immunostimulant to suppress tumors.

ECHINACEA (Echinacea angustifolia)

Resembling a black-eyed Susan, echinacea or purple coneflower is a North American herbaceous perennial that is also called snakeroot because it grows from a thick black root which Indians used to treat snake bites, indicative of the blood-cleansing quality attributed to this herb.

Native American tribes of the Plains States region are known to have used echinacea for medicinal purposes, notably as an antispasmodic or analgesic (pain killer). Indians also used the juice of the plant to bathe burns, the root to treat toothaches and sore throats, as well as for colds and flu. They would sprinkle the herb over a burning fire for "sweats" for purification purposes. During the 1920s, echinacea was one of this country's most popular plant drugs. Herbalists have long appreciated the healing benefits of echinacea as an effective antiviral and as a blood purifier to cure a host of ailments, including rheumatism, psoriasis, dyspepsia, gangrene, tumors, eczema and hemorrhoids.

Echinacea is regarded as a potent immunostimulator and as such has been used to treat such ailments as herpes, infections, candida and cancer. The herb has also been used to help restore normal immune function in cancer patients undergoing chemotherapy.

Studies have shown echinacea prevents the formation of an enzyme which destroys a natural barrier between healthy tissue and damaging organisms, such as herpes and influenza viruses. The herb is the most popular flu and cold remedy in Germany.

ELDERBERRY (Sambucus canadensis)

This herb has been intertwined with human history from the very beginning. Traces of elderberry have been found in Stone Age sites. It provided the wood for Christ's cross. Judas hung himself from an elder tree. Seventeenth century herbalist John Evelyn so highly regarded the elderberry, he called it a remedy "against all infirmities whatever." Gypsies agreed, calling it the "healingest tree on earth." Hippocrates wrote of its value as a purgative. One of Shakespeare's characters referred to it as "the stinking elder." There is even one growing outside of Westminster Abbey, planted there for its mystical ability to ward off evil spirits and disease.

Elder was widely used by several American Indian tribes. The Houmas boiled bark for use as a wash for inflammations. The Menominees used the dried flowers to brew a tea to reduce fevers. And the Meskivakis made tea from the root bark as an expectorant, and to treat headaches. Cooked elderberries were prepared as a drink by some tribes for neuralgia, sciatica and back pain, while others used the leaves in sweat baths to induce profuse sweating which brought relief from rheumatism pain. Scientific evidence exists that a substance in elderberries does in fact stimulate perspiration.

Externally, the herb has been used to relieve skin inflammation such as burns, rashes, and eczema. Elderberries are a good source of vitamins A, B, and C, plus flavonoids.

The berries are also the source of popular elderberry wine, regarded by many as a tonic, and the
cooked berries are main ingredients for pies and jams.
Most recently, new evidence was found to indicate remarkable value in an elderberry extract in the treatment of the flu virus.

EPHEDRA (Ephedra sinica)

This herb goes by the American names of cowboy tea
and squaw tea, reflecting its use by early pioneers and
Mormon settlers who used it primarily for asthma relief. It is also called Mormon tea, since it is brewed as
a pleasant piney substitute for coffee and black tea,
which Mormons avoid. The tea was made from powder
derived from the dried green twigs of the shrub.

The Chinese name for ephedra is ma huang. The
Chinese species of the herb grows in the Inner Mon-
golia region of China. Ephedra has been used in the
Orient for nearly 5,000 years to treat asthma and
upper respiratory symptoms such as coughs, as well as
to reduce fevers and treat allergic skin reactions, such
as hives.

Imported from China and cultivated in dry regions
of North America, ephedra contains an alkaloid called
ephedrine which provides effective decongestant,
bronchodilator, antiasthmatic, and antiallergic functions. A synthetic version of ephedrine called pseudo-
ephedrine is an ingredient found in many over-the-
counter cold and allergy medications.

Ephedra has also been found to promote weight
loss. This is due to its fat-metabolizing ability and to
the fact that it suppresses appetite—an effect that is
enhanced when it is combined with caffeine.

EUCALYPTUS (Eucalyptus globulus)

Native to Australia, where they account for 75 percent
of the vegetation, eucalyptus trees are tall, graceful

trees with slender, silvery leaves and creamy bark. Eucalyptus leaves are the dietary mainstay of koala bears, and humans use eucalyptus oil for a wide variety of medicinal purposes.

It is the aborigines of Australia who were first to discover that eucalyptus oil possesses medicinal properties. The most popular application of eucalyptus oil is for respiratory ailments. Used in a vaporizer, it doesn't take long for the volatile oils to help you breathe more freely and relieve the symptoms of a cold, chronic bronchitis, or asthma.

Eucalyptus oil (eucalyptol) is an effective expectorant used in many commercial drops or lozenges and in liquid preparations to loosen mucus from the nose and lungs and relieve upper respiratory discomfort. Distilled from leaves, the volatile oil is also used as a germicide.

Applied to the skin, eucalyptus oil increases the flow of blood to the area, bringing warming relief from stiffness and swelling, arthritis and rheumatism. The oil also possesses antiseptic qualities useful in the treatment of both respiratory infections and skin diseases. When aged, the oil forms ozone, a form of oxygen that will specifically destroy bacteria, fungi and certain viruses.

FEVERFEW (Chrysanthemum parthenium)

The name of this hardy biennial or perennial herb suggests its early use to bring down a fever. The ancient Greek herbalist, Dioscorides, used the herb to treat arthritis and also believed it helped regulate the uterus during the process of childbirth.

In the lengthy history of this herb, it has been used as an aromatic to ward off disease, for toothaches, as an insect repellent, and against a variety of ailments including kidney stones, constipation, arthritis, infant colic, and vertigo.

Perhaps the most effective modern-day application of feverfew is for headaches, but, as early as 1649, Culpeper noted that feverfew "is very effectual for all pains in the head." Later, in 1772, another famous herbalist, John Hell, wrote, "in the worst headache, this herb exceeds whatever else is known." But it wasn't until 1978 when British newspapers reported that a woman had cured her migraines with feverfew that medical researchers decided to examine the medicinal value of the herb. In 1980, *Lancet,* the highly respected British medical journal, reported that the herb shared properties with aspirin. Then in 1985, the *British Medical Journal* reported another study confirming that feverfew helps alleviate the pain of migraines. Three years later, *Lancet* confirmed the efficacy of feverfew in treating migraines. Once again, pharmaceutical companies have worked feverishly (no pun intended) to isolate the active ingredients of feverfew and turn it into a synthetic patent medicine—but with no success. It is the synergistic combination of ingredients in the feverfew plant that brings on such effective migraine relief.

Feverfew works to inhibit the release of two inflammatory substances—serotonin and prostaglandins—both believed to contribute to the onset of migraine attacks. It also appears that compounds in feverfew serve to make muscle cells less responsive to certain chemicals in the body that trigger migraine muscle spasms. Curiously, feverfew works only for migraines and not regular headaches.

GARLIC (Allium sativum)

Though it is best known as a culinary herb or vampire retardant, the medicinal benefits and claims for garlic are prodigious and worthy of the appellation "wonder drug among all herbs." Throughout recorded history, garlic has been used all over the world for a wide variety of conditions. In folk medicines it has been used for the plague, coughs, tuberculosis, diarrhea, as an antiseptic, to promote kidney function, as a blood cleanser, to kill intestinal parasites, and to prevent heart disease and cancer. It is also used as an antibiotic and antifungal.

Garlic is noted in ancient Chinese writings, mentioned in the Bible and in Homer's *Odyssey*, and has been found in the ancient tombs of Egypt. The Egyptians, incidentally, are said to have fed garlic to the slaves building the Pyramids to give them extra strength and nourishment.

Louis Pasteur discovered that garlic cloves would kill microorganisms in a petri dish. While working as a missionary in Africa, Dr. Albert Schweitzer used garlic to treat cholera, typhus, and amoebic dysentery. During both world wars, before the advent of antibiotics, garlic juice was daubed on infected wounds as a disinfectant to prevent gangrene. The Soviet Army relied so heavily on garlic that it earned the designation "Russian penicillin."

Modern-day research helps explain the broad applications of this "miracle" herb. The same component that gives garlic its strong odor is the one that destroys or inhibits various bacteria and fungi. This component is allicin, which, when garlic is crushed, combines with the enzyme allinase and results in antibacterial action equivalent to one percent penicillin. Garlic is reported to be even more effective than penicillin against typhus disease. It works well against both strep and staph bacteria, and the organisms responsible for cholera, dysentery and enteritis.

The irritating quality of garlic's volatile oil, readily absorbed into the bloodstream, may explain its use for respiratory problems by opening up lungs and bronchial tubes.

On top of everything else it does, this fascinating herb has been found to inhibit tumor cell formation and is under further investigation by the National Cancer Institute for its cancer-inhibiting qualities.

Please be aware that cooking garlic diminishes its potency, but several full-strength supplements and combinations of garlic are commercially available.

GINGER (Zingiber officinale).

It is the knotty branched root of this tropical perennial that is used for medicinal purposes as well as a pungent condiment. The Chinese have used ginger medicinally for well over 2,000 years. It is primarily employed to treat gastrointestinal disorders, particularly the removal of gas, colic, and indigestion. The herb possesses the ability to calm an upset stomach and to stop gripping and cramping in the abdominal and intestinal areas.

Ginger is a very effective and safe antinauseant, acting to prevent the symptoms of motion sickness and "morning sickness" in pregnant women including vomiting, dizziness and cold sweats. Drinking tea containing ginger for colds and asthma has long been a popular American remedy.

Ginger is a mild stimulant, promoting good circulation. Laboratory tests indicate ginger will lower cholesterol levels and inhibit the clotting and aggregation of blood.

A few drops of warmed ginger oil in the ear can soothe earaches. Grated ginger mixed with a little oil and applied to the scalp helps remedy dandruff. Ginger has also been credited with relieving headache and toothache pain.

GINKGO (Ginkgo biloba)

Ginkgo biloba is the Earth's oldest living tree species, traced back more than 200 million years. The tree itself can live 1,000 years, reaching over 100 feet high and 4 feet in diameter. The medicinal use of this "living fossil" goes back nearly 5,000 years.

An extract of ginkgo offers significant benefit to people with impaired blood flow to the brain. Symptoms of this cerebral insufficiency, commonly associated with aging, include short-term memory loss, headache, tinnitus (ringing in the ears), vertigo, and depression. Due to its high flavonoid content, ginkgo also improves circulation throughout the whole body, resulting in an increase in oxygen and blood sugar utilization to all internal organ systems and lower extremeties, thereby addressing problems related to poor circulation such as phlebitis. This positive vascular effect also serves to treat symptoms of underlying arterial insufficiency, providing protection against the development of Alzheimer's disease, strokes and hearing loss. It is a valuable medicine for diabetics, who suffer from impaired circulation to the extremities.

Free radical scavenging and antioxidant effects have been attributed to ginkgo and, hence slowing the process responsible for premature aging and cancer.

Hemorrhoids have been successfully treated by taking ginkgo extract. In one study, 86 percent of patients reported bleeding and pain stopped.

The effects of ginkgo as an antiallergenic and as an antiasthmatic agent have been scientifically demonstrated.

GINSENG (Panax ginseng)

This small perennial herb is without doubt the most famous medicinal plant of China. It was the Chinese who first noted that roots of ginseng resemble the human body and interpreted this as a sign of a medicine that could enhance the whole of human health. A portion that looked like a man would bring a higher price than an entire bale of nondescript roots. The word ginseng literally means "root of man" and the botanical name of one type, panax, is derived from "panacea."

Ginseng has been in use in China for 5,000 years as a tonic and rejuvenator. A Soviet scientist dubbed ginseng an "adaptogen," for its unique ability to normalize or bring into balance whatever is out of balance in the body. For example, if blood sugar levels are low, or if blood pressure is too high, an adaptogen will bring them back to normal levels. Ginseng acts on the pituitary, working to regulate blood sugar, supports the adrenal glands, and generally promotes physical and mental alertness, increasing energy and stamina. Diminishing fatigue is one reason athletes find particular benefit from the use of this herb.

Ginseng is believed to increase women's level of hormones, and is consequently recommended for some women for menopausal symptoms.

The herb stimulates weight and tissue growth and thereby enhances the body's resistance to disease. It particularly benefits the digestive process and the lungs and therefore treats lack of appetite, chronic diarrhea, shortness of breath or wheezing and insomnia.

Studies have shown that ginseng not only inhibits the production of cancer cells, but actually converts the abnormal cells into normal ones.

The hormone-like structure found in ginseng's saponins has a stimulatory action on sexual function in males and females, which may support the herb's reputation for enhancing sexual desire.

GOLDENSEAL (Hydrastis canadensis)

Widely used by a number of Native American tribes, goldenseal is a broad spectrum herb with a reputation for great medicinal virtuosity and, as a result, has been recommended for the treatment of many conditions and ailments.

An infusion of the roots is made into a wash for sore eyes and for skin diseases. Other uses of goldenseal include treatment for indigestion, loss of appetite and liver problems. It has been available as a commercial medicine in North America and throughout Europe for well over a hundred years.

Goldenseal is primarily used to treat congestion and soothe inflammatory conditions of the mucous membranes that line the respiratory, gastrointestinal, digestive, and genitourinary tracts. Goldenseal owes its medicinal value to its high content of the alkaloids hydrastine, hydrastinine and the more well-known gerberine. These alkaloids produce a strong astringent, antibiotic and immune-stimulating effect on mucous membranes.

Antibacterial components in goldenseal have proven effective in the treatment of diarrhea.

One experiment with goldenseal extract on laboratory animals brought about a drop in blood pressure.

Goldenseal can be used as an external application to arms and legs in the treatment of disorders of the lymphatic system and blood vessels. One folk remedy calls for rubbing goldenseal tea on the skin to treat eczema and ringworm.

A component of goldenseal was found to have anticonvulsive effects on the uterus. Goldenseal can also soothe irritated gums, help prevent gum disease and treat canker sores.

The herb is commonly used for female ailments such as vaginitis, and a douche of goldenseal can help relieve fungal infections such as Candida.

HAWTHORN (*Crataegus oxyacantha*)

The brilliant red berries of the hawthorn tree hang in dense clusters from thorny branches and remain on the tree until after the leaves drop in autumn.

Since the 17th century, hawthorn has had a history of use for its positive effects on the cardiovascular system. Traditionally, this herb was involved in the treatment of digestive problems, insomnia, and sore throat. Both Asian and North American cultures used hawthorn for weight loss. It also works as a diuretic, assisting the body in the elimination of excess salt and water.

Hawthorn benefits the heart in three ways: 1) flavonoids in hawthorn work to increase oxygen utilization by the heart, 2) it increases enzyme metabolism and acts as a mild dilator of heart muscle, and 3) it acts as a peripheral vasodilator (dilates blood vessels away from the heart), thereby lowering blood pressure and relieving the burden placed on the heart.

Specific cardiac symptoms for which hawthorn may be called for include recovery from a heart attack, cardiopulmonary disease, high blood pressure, and irregular heartbeat.

Hawthorn in combination with digitalis is given for cardiac problems such as palpitations, angina, and rapid heartbeat (tachycardia). One experiment indicated a mixture of hawthorn and the herb motherwort might prove an effective preventive or treatment for heart disease. Components in hawthorn have been shown to lower cholesterol as well as the size of plaque in arteries.

KAVA KAVA (Piper methysticum)

This herb, a member of the pepper family, grows as a bush in the South Pacific. The first European to discover it was Captain James Cook while he was sailing the South Seas. It was consumed during Polynesian religious rites for its ability to relax and soothe the mind.

Kava is also used for its medicinal effects as a sedative, muscle relaxant, diuretic, and as a remedy for nervousness and insomnia. The herb is also used as a pain reliever and can often be used instead of NSAIDs. (drugs such as aspirin, acetaminophen and ibuprofen).

Studies have shown kava to be as effective in treating anxiety and depression as the prescription antianxiety agents known as benzodiazepines (such as Valium), but without the adverse side effects. In fact, while the benzodiazepines tend to promote lethargy and mental impairment, kava has been shown to improve concentration, memory and reaction time for people suffering from anxiety.

LAVENDER (Lavandula officinalis)

Considered by some to be the quintessential English garden herb, and highly regarded for its classic fragrance in fancy soaps, sachets and potpourris, lavender also is important as a medicinal herb.

Traditionally, the flowers or oil from this old-fashioned herb were used to protect clothes and stored linens from hungry moths. It was also perhaps one of the first air fresheners, often found in early sickrooms. The name "lavender" is actually derived from the Latin verb "to wash," and both Greeks and Romans would scent their baths with the herb. Lavender was an ingredient of aromatic spirits of ammonia, the smelling salts that prevented or relieved fainting spells.

In China, the herb is used in a cure-all oil they call White Flower Oil. It is used as a medicine for hysteria, hoarseness, toothaches, colic, and skin conditions such as eczema and psoriasis. Oil distilled from the perfumy flowers of lavender has applications as a stimulant, a tonic, for headache relief and for relief of intestinal gas. It has also been used to quiet coughs and was once used as a disinfectant for wounds. Applied as a compress, warm lavender tea or oil provides relief for neuralgic pains, rheumatism, sprains, and sore joints.

LICORICE (Glycyrrhiza glabra)

We think of this plant as a candy flavoring (even though most licorice is actually flavored with anise oil); however, the root and constituents of this herb provide a tremendous number of valuable medicinal properties.

Two thousand years ago, the Chinese ranked licorice "superior," which meant it could be used over a long period of time with no toxic effects. They used licorice as a tonic to combat fevers and as a remedy for infection. It is the single most-used herb in Chinese medicine.

Ancient Greeks used licorice as a thirst quencher and to relieve swelling caused by water retention. The Blackfoot Indians used steeped wild licorice leaves in water as an earache remedy. Dutch physicians tested licorice as an aid for indigestion, which led to the use of the herb to treat peptic ulcers.

Other medicinal applications for licorice have included treatment of fever, menstrual and menopausal problems, influenza, arthritis, irritated urinary or bowel passages, and hypoglycemia. Additionally, it has been used as a diuretic, laxative and antispasmodic.

The most common medical use of licorice is for treating upper respiratory ailments including coughs, hoarseness, sore throat, and bronchitis. The rhizomes and roots in licorice have a high mucilage content which, when mixed with water or used in cough drops or syrup, is soothing to irritated mucous membranes and contributes to its use as an expectorant.

Another component of licorice, glycyrrhizin, stimulates the secretion of the adrenal cortex hormone aldosterone, and has a powerful cortisone-like effect. In fact, one study found glycyrrhizin was as effective a cough suppressant as codeine, and safer. In Europe, this unique compound is used extensively for its anti-inflammatory properties, especially for Addison's disease and ulcers. It has exhibited antiviral activity and as a result is used in Japan to treat chronic hepatitis B.

MILK THISTLE (Silybum marianus)

This herb is a stout annual or biennial plant, found in dry, rocky soils. One of the active principles of milk thistle is the flavonoid silymarin, which has been shown to have a direct effect on the cells of the liver, enhancing the overall function of this critical organ.

The known medicinal value of milk thistle is almost exclusively to support the liver. The liver detoxifies poisons that enter the bloodstream, such as alcohol, nicotine, heavy metals (e.g., lead and mercury) and environmental pollutants such as carbon monoxide and pesticides.

To underscore the importance of the liver, it is the source of the bile necessary for the breakdown of fats. It is also where vitamins A, D, E, and K are stored. No wonder the liver is referred to as the body's "chemical factory," and that the silymarin in milk thistle is so important.

In countless scientific studies, silymarin is reported to have shown positive effects in treating nearly every known form of liver disease, including cirrhosis, hepatitis, necroses, and chemical or drug and alcohol-induced liver ailments.

Silymarin's remarkable ability to prevent liver destruction and support liver function is believed to be due to its ability to inhibit the factors responsible for liver damage coupled with the fact it works to stimulate production of new liver cells to replace the old damaged ones. In addition, silymarin acts as an antioxidant, with far greater free radical damage control than even vitamin E in the liver.

Other studies have found that milk thistle offers some protection against the toxic side effects of the pain-relieving drug acetaminophen (Tylenol), a popular analgesic medication.

VITEX/CHASTEBERRY (Vitex agnus castus)

Chasteberry (also called vitex) was at one time recommended as a means for reducing excessive sexual desire, hence the significance of the "chaste" name for the plant. It is for this alleged effect that chasteberry was also used as a spice at monasteries during the Middle Ages where it was called "Monk's pepper."

Traditionally, chasteberry was very popular in Europe as a woman's remedy for regulating the reproductive system, treating PMS and unpleasant side effects associated with menopause, such as hot flashes.

Research has revealed the presence of a volatile oil in chasteberry which tends to balance the production of women's hormones. This oil is believed to contain a progesterone-like substance, which could explain the herb's therapeutic effect in relation to PMS symptoms such as anxiety, nervous tension, insomnia and mood changes, as well as problems associated with menopause such as hot flashes, vaginal dryness, dizziness and depression. Compounds in chasteberry also produce positive results when treating endometriosis, migraines, edema in the legs, cramps, and some allergies. Chasteberry has also been used to treat irregular menstruation, heavy bleeding and fibroid cysts.

Chasteberry extract can also improve skin conditions like acne by balancing sex hormones.

THE MINTS (Mentha)

We're talking here about more than the mint from the garden patch used to freshen a tall glass of lemonade or a mint julep.

All mints have cool, refreshing properties, and they have been used since antiquity all over the world in cooking and for their medicinal value. There are countless varieties and species of mints and all are generally stimulating and relieve indigestion, but three stand out in the herbal medicine cabinet: peppermint, spearmint, and pennyroyal.

Peppermint: The leaves of this perennial are a deeper, richer color than the bright, vivid green of spearmint. This species is also more stimulating to the circulation and is a stronger remedy for alleviating flatulence, heartburn and indigestion. Rather than cool off with a cold beverage in summer, the Chinese refresh themselves with a hot peppermint tea which leaves them feeling cooler because the infusion brings more blood to the skin causing perspiration, which then evaporates away the heat of the body. A stronger tea can be instrumental in breaking a fever. Peppermint is excellent for heartburn, stomach ache, nausea, and migraines.

Among other volatile oils, peppermint contains menthol and therefore has a minor antiseptic quality and is used as a gargle for sore throats and to cleanse wounds. Have a cup of mint tea after a heavy or rich dinner, because menthol also stimulates the flow of bile to the stomach, which promotes digestion and relieves upset stomach.

A simple tea makes a good headache remedy and can be useful to relieve tension and insomnia.

Spearmint: Much like peppermint, spearmint is an aromatic stimulant used for mild indigestion, to cure nausea, relieve stomach spasms and bowel pains, flatulence, motion sickness, and heartburn.

Spearmint tastes different from peppermint, and is also not as strong due to the fact that it contains no menthol. For this reason, spearmint can be substituted for the stronger mint when small children or very old people are being treated.

Pennyroyal: This herb, referred to as the "lung mint," was used to treat coughs and colds. It promotes perspiration to the point it helps break a fever. American Indians utilized pennyroyal to relieve menstrual cramps, and herbalists have recommended this mint to induce menstruation and treat premenstrual syndrome (PMS). Because of its ability to induce menstruation, pennyroyal should not be used by pregnant women. Pennyroyal oil makes an excellent insect repellent for pets.

SAW PALMETTO (Serenoa repens)

Saw palmetto is a small scrubby palm tree native to the U.S. Atlantic coast from South Carolina down through Florida. The tea from the berries of saw palmetto has long been used to treat urinary conditions and has been highly regarded as a remedy for enlarged prostate for centuries. Indeed, saw palmetto was tagged the "plant catheter" due to its therapeutic effect on the neck of the bladder and the prostate in men.

An extract of the saw palmetto will decrease urinary frequency, especially during night, due to inflammation of the bladder and enlargement of the prostate. Reduced urinary flow, dribbling, and impotence are symptomatic of an enlarged prostate or benign prostatic hyperplasia (BPH).

BPH is thought to be caused by a dysfunction of a type of the male hormone testosterone. Saw palmetto extract works to prevent testosterone from converting into dihydrotestosterone, the hormone thought to cause prostate cells to multiply excessively, leading to enlargement of the prostate. It is when the prostate grows abnormally that it pinches the urethra and interferes with urination. Early and effective treatment is important because when the urethra becomes completely blocked, urine can back up into the kidneys, causing severe abdominal pain which calls for immediate medical attention.

Others believe saw palmetto stimulates and increases bladder contractions, which facilitates easier and less painful urine flow.

Preliminary evidence exists to also suggest saw palmetto may also aid those suffering from thyroid deficiency. Moreover, this herb is a good expectorant for use in clearing chest congestion and is used to treat coughs due to colds as well as asthma and bronchitis.

ST. JOHN'S WORT (Hypericum perforatum)

Squeeze the petals of the flower from this shrubby perennial and a blood-colored resin will ooze out, which may explain why, according to legend, this plant sprang from the blood of Saint John the Baptist when he was beheaded.

For centuries in Europe, St. John's wort has been utilized as a mild tranquilizer and a treatment for depression and anxiety. While synthetic psychotropic drugs manufactured to treat these symptoms are associated with significant side effects (constipation, impaired urination, drowsiness), St. John's wort extract at recommended dosages shows no adverse side effects.

St. John's wort is also a muscle relaxant and is used to treat menstrual cramps. It is widely used for insomnia, and in Europe it is a popular remedy for gastrointestinal disorders.

Externally, it is an antiseptic and painkiller for burns and other irritations of the skin. Ointments containing St. John's wort are used to treat rheumatism and sciatica.

Most recently, evidence has surfaced that indicates components in St. John's wort may inhibit the growth of retroviruses in animals, including HIV, the AIDS virus.

TEA TREE OIL (Melaleuca alternifolia)

The tea tree is a small tree native to Australia, where it is acclaimed for its broad medical applications, particularly those affecting the skin. Although used in throat lozenges and in toothpastes, the oil distilled from tea tree leaves is most used externally.

In 1930, a surgeon in Sydney, Australia first noted the positive effect of tea tree oil for cleaning and healing surgical wounds. It has subsequently been determined that tea tree oil exhibits significant antiseptic and antifungal properties as well as stimulating skin rejuvenation.

The established value of tea tree oil as a disinfectant, coupled with the fact that it possesses good penetration properties and is nonirritating, makes it useful for a vast number of conditions including acne, diaper rash, heat rash, athlete's foot, canker sores, corns, insect bites, ringworm, lice, mouth ulcers, boils, sore throat, burns, psoriasis, root canal treatment, dandruff, respiratory congestion, gingivitis, herpes and yeast infections.

Tea tree oil is available in many products such as toothpastes, shampoos, soaps, throat lozenges, hair conditioners and skin lotions, and is packaged in forms such as salves, ointments, gels and liniments. Use as directed on the label.

UVA URSI (*Arctostaphylos uva ursi*)

The leaves of this perennial ground cover, known as bearberry, have an extended record as a folk remedy, particularly in relation to urinary tract problems. It is said that the Chinese introduced Marco Polo to this herb when he was traveling in China. European herbalists in the 13th century recognized the healing benefits of uva ursi.

Before the development of synthetic diuretic and urinary antiseptic drugs, uva ursi leaves were the main medicine available for these applications. The Chinese, European, and American natives all adopted uva ursi as an herb for healing the kidneys, using the leaves and fresh berries for treating kidney stones, bladder infections, and incontinence. Some tribes also mixed uva ursi leaves with other herbs and honey as a longevity elixir.

The strong urinary antiseptic, diuretic and astringent qualities of uva ursi are attributable to the active constituents hydroquinone and arbutin, which, interestingly, possess a more potent effect working together than either acting separately.

Analysis has shown that uva ursi contains a substance known to soothe and speed repair of irritated tissues. The herb has also exhibited antiviral, antibacterial and antifungal as well as antiplaque actions.

WHITE WILLOW BARK (*Salix alba*)

The white willow was introduced into the United States from Europe, and is now found gracing rivers and streams throughout the country. The bark is the part of the willow used medicinally and is easily removed in the spring when the sap begins to flow.

Willows have been tapped since antiquity for pain relief and reduction of fever. Ancient manuscripts of Egypt, Greece, and Assyria refer to willow bark, and even Hippocrates recommended willow to counter pain.

People have chewed the leaves or the inner bark of willows in this family of plants for thousands of years, and all contain salicylic acid. This compound was originally used by the Bayer Company in Germany in the late 1890s to synthesize acetylsalicylic acid, otherwise known as aspirin.

Natural salicylic acid is nearly as potent as aspirin. However, the compound salicin from willow does not cause gastric or intestinal upset of bleeding as aspirin can. This is because the natural product does not block prostaglandins in the stomach or intestines.

WITCH HAZEL (Hamamelis virginiana)

Witch hazel is a name derived from an old English word for "pliant," and the branches of this deciduous tree are in fact limber and were used as archery bows. Witch hazel is used principally as a skin liniment and astringent. Available in extract form, its anti-inflammatory action helps soothe minor scrapes, cuts and bruises. Applied externally to varicose veins or hemorrhoids, it helps relieve the pain and itching that accompany these conditions. A decoction of the bark is used as a dandruff wash, and the extract is useful for insect bites and sunburn.

PART III
Growing and Using the Healing Herbs

CHAPTER 6

Preparing and Taking Herbs

Just the slightest crush releases the wonderful aromas of plants like mint in our gardens and kitchens. This is one of the simplest ways to sample the powerful essence of herbs, one we use all the time in our kitchens. Freshly chopped mint with our potatoes or dandelion leaves in salad are examples of how it's often easy to take herbs as food. Frequently, though, it's more convenient or appropriate to use a herbal preparation. Then the trick is to capture the essence in usable forms. The range of herbal preparations is wide, including, for example, ointments for external application and capsules to be swallowed.

However an herb is prepared, its effect is achieved by interaction with our body chemistry. The aim is to ensure absorption and uptake by the bloodstream. Once circulating in the blood, an herb exerts its specific influence on the body. The key to traditional use and the work of skilled herbalists has always been the use of an herb's effects to support the body's own natural efforts to recover. This is unlike the tendency of many modern drugs designed to suppress the body's responses and produce short-term comfort.

This is not to say herbs can't bring immediate relief, as anyone who has soothed sunburn with aloe or calmed a toothache with oil of cloves will tell you. It is more that herbal treatments are gentler and aligned to the body's own processes. Treatment of illness with herbs may well require a little more time than a "knock-'em-dead" blast say, of antibiotics, but will be without the same risk of side effects and with much more likelihood of tackling the root cause.

Different conditions suit different methods of treatment based on selection of the best route for absorption of the herb. Absorption can take place through the digestive system, the skin, the lining of the mouth, ear and the nose, as with inhalation of hot vapors. Herbs are widely available now in a diversity of forms. Best results are obtained from organically grown fresh herbs. They should be preserved by proper drying and storage, so always check the source and avoid pills packed with fillers.

Many preparations can also be homemade, although the strongest form, essential oils, are best bought. Review the choices and enjoy tailoring your selection to your own particular needs. Remember—use herbs as directed, following the same precautions as with any medicine and always consult your physician if you are already being treated for a condition.

DROPS AND SPOONFULS

Some of the best internal herbal preparations are liquid and include syrups and tinctures. Tinctures are preservative mixtures of the herb in alcohol and water. Alcohol not only helps herbs last longer, it is also a good solvent for many of their active components. A standard ratio is 1:5 of the herb to the fluid. An example would be 7 ounces (200 grams) of herbs to 4½ cups (1 liter) of alcohol such as vodka, although cider vinegar can be used instead if preferred. For homemade tinctures, place the herbs in a dark, screw-top jar and cover them with the alcohol. The mixture should be shaken twice daily and stored, tightly covered, in a warm place. Use a muslin cloth to strain the residue, squeezing well, after two weeks. Tightly stoppered dark bottles help prevent evaporation and destruction of constituents by light.

Tinctures are usually taken with water and are a very concentrated way to take herbs. Some people like to add them to teas or even compresses. Mixing a tincture with a little beeswax, cocoa butter, or olive oil is also a useful way to make an ointment. And syrups? These are in fact tinctures added to sugar—a sweet way to make the herb go down!

A NICE CUP OF HERB

Drinking herbal teas can be one of the most pleasurable and effective ways of getting herbs into your system, although the taste of some leaves a lot to be desired! Teas are actually infusions. Boiling water helps extract and dissolve some of the medicinal compounds of an herb. This is a particularly useful way to prepare herbs desired for their potent aromatic oils, compounds which give teas their strong aromas. Tea bags or tea leaves are made from the dried herb and are generally equivalent to three parts of the fresh plant. When no particular dose is sought, a herbal tea can become more of a tonic, or included as part of a remedy, rather than one on its own.

Whereas infusions mainly use the soft, above-ground parts of plants, decoctions are another method of producing drinkable herbs. Decoctions are usually made with the woodier parts of plants like roots and bark. The chopped herb is brought to boil for 10 to 15 minutes, then strained immediately. More volatile components are lost, but decoctions capture the mineral salts and bitter principles, which can lead to some "interesting" tastes and powerful healing!

TAKE ONE AS DIRECTED

Some herbal preparations are in capsule form, as with many supplements and medicines. Gelatin containers are filled with finely powdered herbs, oils or extracted juice, usually in a hypoallergenic form. On reaching the gut, the shell is broken down, releasing the contents for absorption.

Herbs also come in traditional pill, tablet or lozenge form. Mucilage, gum, dry sugar or other binders and fillers are mixed with the powdered herb or with oil to make tablets or lozenges. Lozenges can be sucked, allowing them to be taken by a small degree into the bloodstream directly through the blood vessels of the mouth, but largely, again, through the walls of the intestine.

Homeopathic and some other preparations of herbs involve solutions mixed with sugar bases to create small pills. These are then placed under the tongue where they dissolve. This is known as sub-lingual absorption and is useful because it bypasses the liver. Always hungry to fuel its own processes, the liver is the blood's first major "stop" on its route from the stomach, and it is sometimes helpful to direct absorption elsewhere first.

APPLY WITH CARE, RUB GENTLY . . .

Many conditions are relieved by direct absorption of herbs through the skin. Sometimes part of the plant itself is used as with fresh aloe or mugwort, rubbed onto skin troubled by poison oak. Tinctures in fatty or oily bases make ointments, while more fluid liniments are herb extracts mixed with oils or alcohol.

Herbs can also be wrapped in material to make poultices which are laid on the skin. You can make compresses with wads of material soaked in herb decoctions or infusions. Topical applications like these are very useful for treating localized conditions like cuts, sprains and aches.

Expert massage can also involve specific herbal treatments with extracts of essential plant oils as in aromatherapy. The general benefits of a good all-over rub with a perfumed oil have been recognized for centuries. There's also nothing like relaxing in a bath of herbal salts as a way to feel the benefits of herbs working from the outside in.

GREAT HERB COMBOS

On the herbalist's menu are many formulas or combinations of medicinal plants established over history as stronger or broader in their effects than treatment with a single herb. Passionflower and valerian are good examples. Both reduce tension and anxiety, and a combination produces a double action, a natural sedative for short-term use.

Scientific investigation goes on to prove the synergistic value of combining herbs, balancing or increasing their individual chemical effects. For instance, sedative herbs are often supported by more stimulating ones like damiana to enable the body chemistry to even out rather than to swing one particular way. Licorice is used with the laxatives senna and cascara. The latter can cause intestinal pain, but licorice, itself a mild laxative, contains anti-inflammatory chemicals and lowers stomach acid levels, thus protecting against the harsher effects of the other two herbs.

Herbal formulas used in this way help to achieve harmony in the body and make very effective remedies.

CHAPTER 7

Your Herbal First Aid Kit for the Home

Herbal Preparation	Disorder	Treatment
Arnica ointment, Arnica tincture	Sprains and bruises, burns, scalds, stings, and impetigo	Rub ointment gently onto unbroken skin or apply a compress of tincture
Calendula tincture, Calendula ointment	Minor cuts	Bathe with tincture and/or apply ointment to cut.
Echinacea tincture	Insect bites	Apply tincture to bite and take one dropperful in water.
Echinacea and goldenseal mixture	Infections, flu and common cold	2-4 dropperfuls in water every 4 waking hours.
Herbal throat spray (with echinacea, goldenseal, and licorice, plus)	Sore throat	Spray back of throat as indicated on container.

Herbal Preparation	Disorder	Treatment
Ginger tea	Nausea	3-4 cups daily.
Peppermint tea	Headaches	3-4 cups daily.
Tea tree oil	Toothache, gum and fungal infections	Apply oil to affected area.
Valerian root tincture	Insomnia	Take drops with water as directed on container.
White willow capsules	Headaches	1 capsule as needed.

CHAPTER 8

Healing Herbs You Can Grow in Your Home or Garden

"The fresher the better" is certainly true of herbs. Gathering from the wild is still possible, but should only be done with an expert guide and with care not to exhaust an area of any one plant. Indoor and outdoor cultivation at your own home can be an enjoyable and inexpensive way to create your own supply of healing and culinary herbs. Starting with seeds gives you a choice of many varieties and is much cheaper than buying the plants themselves. Several herbs make natural partners, repelling insects for example, or promoting plant health, so be alert to opportunities for companion planting.

In tending herbs, you will be following a worldwide, centuries-old tradition. With your own flowerpots or a garden and rich organic soil, you can grow your own mini-pharmacy and reap the benefits of better health, not to mention more flavorful food! Try your hand with some of the herbs listed below and consult organic gardening books for tips on organic soil preparation, pest and disease control, plant layout and propagation.

HERB OR WEED?

Remember to check if a "weed" is itself a useful herb, like dandelion, that is worth cultivating where it will not smother other plants. However, plants such as bindweed, couch grass, creeping buttercup, ground elder and creeping thistle are all best removed as soon as they appear. They're also no good for composting.

HARVEST TIME

Many are the witch's brews that call for strange herbs picked at dawn or by the light of the moon. Actually, both seemingly strange practices make scientific sense because many of the medicinal compounds found in plants are volatile. This means they are evaporated by the sun's heat, so they are at their greatest concentration in plants before the sun is high in the sky. If you can, pick your herbs as soon as the dew has evaporated.

LEAVES AND FLOWERS

Pick leaves and flowers early in the morning, being careful not to bruise them. Flowers are usually best harvested as soon as possible after they have fully opened. For culinary purposes, leaves can be picked any time from a green and healthy plant. For medicinal purposes, however, leaves are usually best collected when flowers are in bud and before any have fully opened. Remember to shake off any insects.

GETTING TO THE ROOTS

Roots contain their greatest concentration of useful substances at the end of the growing season. Collect them at this time, discarding any that are damaged at all. Do not soak roots before drying, but wash them thoroughly to remove all soil.

DRYING HERBS

Always dry your harvest in the shade to avoid extreme temperatures. Try to disturb the plants as little as possible, although herbs dried on paper or trays will need to be turned occasionally. Small quantities can be dried on sheets of paper in a well-ventilated closet or on baking trays in a cool oven with the door open. For larger amounts, a warm, airy and shady space is needed. Herbs can be dried flat on large sheets of paper or on nets or stretched muslin. String up bunches of herbs well away from walls.

Dry small roots whole, but cut large ones into two or more pieces lengthwise. Thread root pieces on a string and hang them up to dry. Remove the outer coat of bulbs and slice before drying. When collecting bark, scrape off the outer layer, then peel away the inner layers, which can be dried in sunlight (except black cherry which needs shade). Temperatures should be *no higher* than 85-95° F for plants and leaves, 115° F for roots and 100° F for bulbs.

Leaves and stems are considered to be dry when they are brittle, breaking readily. Petals are ready when they rustle but do not crumble. Thick roots will chip with a small hammer, but most will snap. Three to seven days is a rough guide for most herbs, which will weigh about one-eighth of the fresh plant weight, but still smell and taste very much like it.

STORING HERBS

Herbs like tarragon, marjoram and thyme can be kept whole for bouquets garnis. Bay leaves, too, are good whole in soups and stews. Small flowers are also best kept intact, although marigold petals can be pulled off if preferred. With stalks removed, crush your dried

herbs with a rolling pin or grinder or use a sieve for
feathery herbs like dill.

Herbs deteriorate when exposed to oxygen and/or
light. For this reason they must be stored in airtight,
opaque containers. Dark glass jars with tight-fitting lids
are best. For everyday use, keep small quantities in
separate containers to lessen the exposure of your
main stock to air and light. Don't forget to label each
container, and dating them is a good idea, too. Keep
herbs in a dark, cool closet or cupboard.

SOME FAVORITE HOME-GROWN
HEALING HERBS

ALOE (Aloe spp.)

Type: Perennial. Many species. **Soil and situation:** Average, well-drained, full sun to light shade. **Spread/
Height:** Up to several feet spread, up to 2 feet height,
with very long stems. **Propagation:** From suckers or
offshoots removed when 1-2 inches on indoor plant,
6-8 inches on outdoor plant. **Flower:** Yellow/orange-
red, tubular, on stalks along a stem. **Leaves:** Pale, gray-
ish-green, rubbery, long, spiky. **Harvest:** Older, outside leaves.

Aloe requires a minimum temperature of around
41°F and is frequently grown as a pot plant indoors,
where it can thrive for years. When propagating, it's
often best to dig up the plant, remove the suckers and
then re-pot. Keeping a pot on the kitchen windowsill
provides a simple remedy for minor burns and cuts
and is always handy. Use scissors to cut off the end of
a leaf, slice it down the middle and scrape out the
clear gel. The gel is wonderfully soothing and is also
used to help heal sunburn, itching and rashes. Aloe
is a major constituent of many skin and hair prepara-

tions, but fresh aloe produces the best results. Josephine, wife to the emperor Napoleon, used a milk-and-aloe lotion to preserve her complexion. Indeed, aloe is said to help clear oily and acned skin. Some find aloe slightly drying, but mixing with a little vitamin E may prevent this.

CATNIP (Nepeta cataria)

Type: Perennial. **Soil and situation:** Average, well-drained, full sun to partial shade. Sow: Difficult with tiny seeds—see "propagation." **Height:** 1-3 feet **Propagation:** 4-inch stem sections rooted in moist medium. **Flower:** Small, tubular, white with purple-pink spots, massed in spikes, summer. **Leaves:** Oval, tooth-edged, gray-green with downy underside. **Harvest:** Tops and leaves when in full bloom.

Cats seem to get quite a high from the aroma of this plant, but don't go looking for the same effect on yourself—our brains are wired to respond differently to the chemicals in catnip! This mild herb, listed in the *U.S. Pharmacopoeia* from 1842 to 1882, has long been used to treat illness in children. Brewed as a hot infusion, catnip promotes sweating and is good for infectious diseases such as measles as well as colds and flu. Soothing to the nervous system, it helps restless children get to sleep. This may be because the chemical structure of a major part of catnip's volatile oil is related to valepotriates, the known sedatives found in valerian. Catnip also has a calming effect on the stomach, and is helpful for colic, flatulence and diarrhea. Its sharp flavor made catnip an ingredient in Roman salads, and catnip tea was very popular in England before foreign varieties cornered the market.

EVENING PRIMROSE (Oenothera biennis)

Type: Biennial. Many other species. **Soil and situation:** Stony, dry, full sun. **Sow:** Late summer. **Spread/**

Height: 2 x 5 feet. **Flower:** Mid-late summer, on spikes, large, bright yellow. **Leaves:** Shiny, long, pointed. **Harvest:** Flowers, seeds, root.

Studies have given substantial support to the use of evening primrose in treating a number of disorders, from dry eyes and brittle nails to hyperactivity in children, premenstrual syndrome, alcoholic poisoning, acne, overweight, rheumatoid arthritis, and coronary artery disease. Evening primrose is very high in essential fatty acids, especially one called GLA which is needed for the production of a hormone-like substance, PGE1, which has a range of beneficial effects in the body. The whole plant is edible. Try a tincture, or infusions can be made with 1 teaspoon of the plant to one cup of water to be taken, one mouthful at a time, once a day. Exercise caution, though, as evening primrose is not recommended for epileptics, and some people have reported sensitivities to the plant.

FENNEL (Foeniculum vulgare)

Type: Semi-hardy perennial. **Soil and situation:** Very well-drained, full sun. **Sow:** Mid-summer, fall. **Spread/ Height:** 3 × 4-6 feet. **Flower:** Small, yellow, on umbrella of stalks, midsummer. **Leaves:** Deep green, thin, feathery, aromatic. **Harvest:** Ripe seeds, young leaves, green stems.

Take care of fennel, for it is vulnerable to harm from certain plants including wormwood, which can inhibit seed germination and stunt its growth, while coriander will prevent seeds from forming. You should also make this herb a loner in your garden because it can damage other plants like bush beans, caraway, tomatoes and kohlrabi. Fennel, with its refreshing anise-like flavor, has long been known as a digestive aid included in recipes by the Greeks, Romans and Anglo-Saxons before spreading even further abroad.

Add fennel to soups and salads. Drink fennel tea for indigestion and heartburn and serve it to babies to relieve their colic. It's also an ancient remedy used to promote the flow of milk in nursing mothers. Fennel eyewash is recommended for tired, sore eyes and the oil is antispasmodic and antibacterial, although not recommended for those with allergies or skin sensitivities.

GARLIC (Allium sativum)

Type: Perennial bulb. Many varieties. **Soil and situation:** Well drained, rich to medium, full sun to partial shade. **Height:** 1 foot. **Propagation:** Split into cloves. Plant early spring or fall. **Flower:** Very small, white to pinkish, late summer. **Leaves:** Long, flat, pointed. **Harvest:** Leaves, early summer; bulbs, late summer.

Many gardeners believe roses benefit from garlic planted close by and, of course, they're a good idea if you're having trouble with vampires! In reality garlic wards off many diseases. Research shows that eating garlic protects against heart disease by lowering cholesterol and other fats, and by reducing blood-clotting activity and hypertension. Garlic is also good for intestinal infections. Take grated garlic mixed with honey for coughs. Apply garlic to wounds to prevent infections. Of course, you can also enjoy garlic's unique flavor in foods.

GERMAN CHAMOMILE (Matricaria chamomilla)

Type: Annual. **Soil and situation:** Most types, especially light. **Sow:** Late summer/fall. **Spread/Height:** 4 inches x 2 feet. **Flower:** From early summer, small, daisy-like. **Leaves:** Feathery, bright green. **Harvest:** Flowers when fully open.

This plant is known as the "doctor's physician" and is described by Germans as "capable of anything." An aid to plants, too, German chamomile repels flying insects and even helps improve onion crop yield. Chamomile flowers contain a lovely blue volatile oil called azulene, and its many effective compounds include two powerful antiseptics. Use externally for hair care, especially fair hair, in combination with soapwort. You can also steep 3-4 ounces in boiling hot water for 1 hour to make a relaxing bath mixture. Make a tincture for washes or compresses to soothe and aid the healing of rashes, burns and wounds.

Brew an infusion and drink chamomile as tea. This will aid nervous conditions, insomnia and neuralgia. Chamomile has also been shown to calm restless children. In fact, chamomile was the tea served to Peter Rabbit by his mother to soothe his aching stomach! It's a famous remedy for digestive upsets, including diarrhea and flatulence, with research proving it is anti-inflammatory, and antispasmodic. Chamomile is also used to prevent and treat ulcers.

GINGER (*Zingiber officinale*)

Type: Tropical biennial. **Soil and situation:** Container, indoors. Loam, sand, peat moss and compost in equal parts. Light shade, warmth, moisture and humidity. **Height:** 2-4 feet. **Propagation:** From rhizome. **Flower:** Rarely in cultivation. Dense spikes, yellow-green, purple spotted and striped. **Leaves:** Grass-like, long, pointed. **Harvest:** Root, 8-12 months after planting.

Ginger is a commercial crop throughout the tropics, supplying an international trade in culinary spices and herbal medicines that goes back thousands of years. For your own harvest, pull the mature plant from its pot, cut off the leafstalks and thinner, fibrous roots. Cut off as much of the main root as you can store and use. The remainder can be re-planted. Wrap your ginger first in a paper towel, then tightly in plastic wrap. Refrigerated, ginger will last for several months. Chew on a fresh stick to relieve a sore throat. Dry some, too, for dry ginger has slightly different chemical actions, traditionally making it more suitable for respiratory and digestive disorders.

All ginger is warming, but fresh ginger induces sweating and is said to be better for treating colds.

Studies have shown ginger provides much relief from nausea in early pregnancy at just 250 milligrams four times daily, and also from the pain, swelling and stiffness of both osteo- and rheumatoid arthritis, using doses from 500 to 4,000 mg daily. Cook Indian style and you'll soon exceed these doses! Daily amounts of 8 to 10 grams are regularly consumed in India where this herb continues to be very popular in both main dishes like curry and desserts such as crystallized ginger.

LAVENDER (Lavandula officinalis)

Type: Perennial shrub, evergreen. **Soil and situation:** Light, well-drained, calcareous, full sun. **Sow:** Early spring or fall without heat. **Spread/Height:** 2 x 2 feet 8 inches. **Propagation:** Spring—softwood cuttings, fall—hardwood cuttings. **Flower:** Mid-summer, mauve. **Leaves:** Narrow, gray-green. **Harvest:** Flowers, mid/late summer.

Use lavender for hedging and cut it back when it has finished flowering. Lavender takes its name from the Latin verb "to wash" and was used by Romans and Greeks to create relaxing, scented baths. Widely known for its lovely scent, lavender is also used in steam inhalation against coughs, colds and chest infections. Make an infusion of lavender for the same conditions as well as for tension, anxiety, stomach and headaches. The oil is antibacterial, helpful for healing cuts, and is one of the best remedies for stings and burns. A few drops used in massage help to relax muscles and ease pain. As with all plant oils, do not take lavender oil internally.

LEMON BALM (Melissa officinalis)

Type: Perennial, evergreen. **Soil and situation:** Average, well-drained, sun or semi-shade. **Sow:** Late spring. **Spread/Height:** 2 feet x 2 feet 8 inches. **Propagation:** In spring, layering, root division, cuttings. **Flower:** Small, white to pink or yellowish, in clusters, summer. **Leaves:** Broad, oval, toothedged, lemon fragrance. **Harvest:** Leaves and stems in growing season.

Lemon balm is a good bee plant, its official name coming from the Greek word for "bees." Strangely, it is also considered to be a good insect repellent, used to keep flies off food and away from fires.

Harvest this herb by cutting off the entire plant two inches above the ground. It needs to be dried within two days of harvesting for it can quickly turn black. A tip from Shakespeare's *Merry Wives of Windsor* is to rub lemon balm into wood, letting its fragrant oils act as a natural equivalent to lemon-scented furniture polish. You can also make a pleasant tea with this herb as a remedy for colds, flu, depression, headache and indigestion. In fact, lemon balm has been recommended for centuries because "it makes the heart merry."

Analysis shows the effects of the plant's volatile oils are due to antispasmodic and strong sedative properties which also make lemon balm helpful for promoting menstrual periods and relieving menstrual cramping. Its polyphenols may be responsible for its antiviral effects, demonstrated against mumps and other viruses. Relax in a cleansing, steamy bath mixture of lemon balm and use it as an acne rinse. Chop it up for culinary use, too, with salads, chicken and lamb. Drink the liqueurs, Benedictine and Chartreuse and you'll be downing lemon balm, too!

MEADOWSWEET (Filipendula ulmaria)

Type: Perennial. **Soil and situation:** Moist, rich, sun or semi-shade. **Sow:** Spring or fall. **Spread/Height:** 1 x 2-3 feet. **Propagation:** Divide roots in spring. **Flower:** Summer, cream, clustered. **Leaves:** Dark green. **Harvest:** Flower heads, leaves, roots in the fall.

Meadowsweet is a good plant to grow by water. Its active compounds include substances like those found in aspirin, antioxidants, vitamin C and sugar. Science shows us how meadowsweet's particular chemical package made it a safe remedy for hundreds of years for conditions like children's diarrhea, rheumatism and fevers. Its anti-inflammatory constituents on their own could cause gastric bleeding, yet it also contains tannin and mucilage which seem to act as buffers, preventing the adverse effect. Meadowsweet also acts as an antiseptic diuretic, aiding the excretion of uric acid. Make a hot infusion to induce sweating, an old-fashioned but useful treatment for fevers. Boil two tablespoons of the plant or dried rootstock in one cup of water and take one cup a day as a remedy. You can also use this decoction as a wash for wounds or sore eyes.

PARSLEY (Petroselinum crispum)

Type: Biennial. **Soil and situation:** Rich, moist, well-drained, sun to semi-shade. **Sow:** Spring inside, warm. Mid-summer outside, full sun with shelter. **Spread/Height:** 1 foot 4 inches x 2 feet. **Propagation:** Allow to self-seed. **Flower:** Tiny, greenish yellow in umbrella clusters, summer. **Leaves:** Dark green, feathery. **Harvest:** Leaves, seeds, root.

You may know that parsley is a useful breath sweetener, but you probably haven't heard how it used to be sprinkled on corpses as a deodorizer! Its high chlorophyll content helps it eat up internal odors (including garlic), and its oils are naturally aromatic, leading to its popular use in bouquets garnis and as a garnish. Parsley is said to be good in a vegetable patch because it is supposed to repel some insects.

An excellent source of vitamin C, usefully packaged with iron, a nibble of parsley makes sense when you're under the weather. You'll also be taking in several B vitamins, vitamin A, calcium, manganese and phosphorus. Its role as a nutritional mini-powerhouse backs up its medicinal effects as a diuretic suitable for treating urinary infections and fluid retention. Because it helps expel uric acid, parsley is a remedy for gout and the root has laxative properties.

Pregnant women should avoid large amounts of parsley. On the other hand, the chemistry of parsley strengthens uterine muscles and increases breast milk. Parsley is a digestive aid and as a tincture, two to 15 drops in water, as needed, it makes a treatment for nausea. Cosmetically, parsley infusions are soothing and cleansing and can be used as a hair rinse. Parsley oil is found in many cosmetics, shampoos, soaps and skin lotions. If you can, freeze your parsley as this is said to give better results than simply drying.

ROSEMARY *(Rosmarinus officinalis)*

Type: Perennial shrub. Many decorative subspecies. **Soil and situation:** Calcareous, well drained, full sun, sheltered from wind. **Sow:** 75-80°F in seed tray. **Height:** 5 feet 8 inches. **Propagation:** From early summer, cuttings of non-flowering shoots. **Flower:** Late spring, pale to deep blue. **Leaves:** Leathery, thin, gray-green, oily, aromatic. **Harvest:** Leaves as needed.

Rosemary's traditional companion is sage. Plant it with carrot, too, as it repels carrot fly. It is an excellent hair tonic, and its refreshing scent leads to its use in cosmetics and perfumes. Ancient Greeks even made rosemary garlands to strengthen their memories at exam times! Medicinally, rosemary has many uses and is listed officially in the *U.S. Pharmacopoeia*. Even as recently as World War II, French hospitals burned juniper berries with rosemary leaves to kill germs. The oil, which, like many essential oils, is antifungal and antibacterial, is part of several liniments for rheumatism and can be applied directly to the head to relieve headaches. Enjoy rosemary with, say, a dish of lamb, and you will be reducing flatulence, stimulating your digestion, liver, gall bladder and circulation. Infusions of rosemary, of course, are used for the same reasons, as well as for treating painful menstruation. Use caution with rosemary, for the undiluted oil should not be taken internally.

SAGE *(Salvia officinalis)*

Type: Perennial shrub. **Soil and situation:** Well-drained, calcareous, full sun. **Sow:** Late spring. **Spread/Height:** 1 foot 8 inches × 1-2 feet. **Propagation:** Cuttings, spring. **Flower:** Tubular, purple, pink, blue or white, early summer. **Leaves:** Gray-green, velvety, aromatic. **Harvest:** Leaves.

Sage is a beneficial companion plant in general and especially for rosemary and vines. In addition, it repels cabbage moths and a number of other harmful flying insects. American Indians used the fragrant, silver-green sagebrush of the American chaparral as a toothbrush, cleanser and remedy with bear grease for skin sores, but its bitter taste rules it out of competition with the cultivated Mediterranean variety for culinary use.

Named from the Latin "to save," sage has been associated for centuries with longevity. The Chinese would even trade up to four times their fine green tea for European sage. As you stuff that turkey, you're dispensing a long-esteemed remedy for sore throats, colds, indigestion, hot flashes and painful periods. Mix sage tea with a little cider vinegar for relief from throat disorders like tonsillitis. Use the tea as a mouthwash for infected gums and mouth ulcers. Feel its volatile oil work as it boosts digestion. It will also stop sweating and is reputed to dry up the flow of breast milk. Sage is also used for treating amenorrhea and painful periods.

This wide range of applications has its origins in the variety of substances found in sage. Besides its powerful oils, sage contains estrogenic compounds, antibacterial agents, antioxidants and tannins. Do note, though, that sage should only be taken as remedy for a week or two at a time, since it has another substance, thujone, which can have potentially toxic effects. But when you turn to sage in the kitchen, remember its extensive medicinal powers as you use it in dishes from soups and salads to meats, cheese and bread.

SWEET BASIL (ocimum basilicum)

Type: Tender annual. One of many varieties. **Soil and situation:** Fertile loam, sun. **Sow:** Spring inside, warm. Midsummer outside, full sun with shelter. **Spread/Height:** 1 × 1-2 feet. **Propagation:** Cuttings. **Flower:** Mid to late summer, white/purplish. **Leaves:** Delicate, clear green, aromatic. **Harvest:** Leaves as needed, stems before flowering.

The chopped leaves of basil are famous for their distinctive flavor in dishes like pesto. Its other main use is as an insect repellent! In Europe, it is grown in pots outside doors to deter flies. Plant it near tomatoes for the same reason. Basil is also recommended for gastric disorders such as stomach cramps and constipation. Steep 1 teaspoon of dried herb in ½ cup of water. Take 1-1½ cups a day, one mouthful at a time. You can even do as some residents of New Mexico and carry basil in your pockets to attract money!

CHAPTER 9

Aromatherapy Herbs

Has a whiff of something ever sent you back to childhood, a special occasion or the company of someone special? Such is the power of smell, harnessed even as a marketing tool, supermarkets creating the illusion of fresh bakeries and real estate agents filling vases, heating vanilla in the oven and brewing coffee! In plants, the source of their potent scents is essential oils. Such oils serve them as insect repellents or attractants, antibacterial and antifungal agents and often lends them a particular character. In perfumes, ointments and sprays they do the same for us! Essential oils act as stimulants or relaxants to humans, frequently providing a link from the physical to the emotional as the olfactory organs connect to the parts of the brain associated with emotions. Formal research is scant, but work done at Milan University gives scientific support to the observation that plant oils can lift our spirits, relieving anxiety and depression.

BREATHE DEEPLY AND RELAX

As volatile substances, plant oils are extracted by distillation or soaking. The result is highly concentrated products which are absorbed through the skin or, diluted, through inhalation. Direct, external use of essential oils dates back thousands of years to ancient Egypt and Greece, and the Far East. Hippocrates en-

73

couraged the burning of aromatic plants to prevent
the spread of plague in ancient Athens. Gattefossé,
an early French aromatherapist, recounted how, on
impulse, he thrust his burnt hand into a bowl of lavender essence and found it healed extremely rapidly.

Today, we can choose an incense to burn, buy commercial vaporizers and visit steam baths. Do-it-yourself
inhalation methods include mixing one or two drops
of essential oil in a bowl of steaming hot water, then
placing a towel over your head and around the bowl
to catch the steam. Soak in a bath, too, where five or
six drops have been dissolved in warm water.

Five or six drops of oil are appropriate for massage,
the oils being diluted in two to five teaspoons of car-
rier oil such as almond, grape seed or soy. Massage
with essential oils stimulates blood circulation, boost-
ing their absorption. It also activates nerve endings,
which aromatherapists believe then channel a reaction
along nerves to the pituitary gland. The pituitary
gland regulates the function of other glands, including the adrenals, and in this way influences whether
we feel stressed or relaxed. This ties in with scientific
analysis of several oils showing them to contain substances known to be stimulative or sedative in their
effects.

Different oils are also reputed to produce different
emotional effects, basil bringing cheer, catnip and rue
inducing calm, and ylang ylang promoting sex and
love, for example. Seek out *natural* essential oils. Keep
in mind that natural oils are very highly concentrated
and pack the power of the plant in a way synthetics
cannot match. Choose your oil to suit, then pamper
yourself with aromatherapy, one of the oldest health
promotion measures known.

CHAPTER 10

Herbs for the Bath

For a wonderful addition to any bath, simply add a few drops of oil or a pint or so of a very strong infusion, strained, of your chosen herb to the bath water. One of the best and simplest herbal bath remedies is eucalyptus. Just on its own, this antiseptic herb brings relief from aches and pain, clears the head and sinuses and warms the body as it increases blood flow. You can also make an herb sachet to soak in the bath and smooth over your skin. Mix two cups of dried flowers, such as lime or chamomile, with one cup of fine oatmeal. Place them in the center of a piece of muslin about 16 inches square. Gather up the edges of the muslin, tying it up tightly with thread or string. Enjoy at least a ten-minute soak with herbal mixtures like those below.

SKIN SAVERS

To soothe dry, itchy or inflamed skin, try a bath mixture with a cold-pressed vegetable oil base. As well as relieving symptoms and helping to protect your skin, such oils provide a natural barrier to moisture loss. Avoid using corn or cottonseed oils as these are derived from crops usually heavily sprayed with pesticides and fungicides. Also avoid mineral oils, as they clog pores. Mix ½ cup of each of almond, safflower, soy, and sesame oils. Shake all these together with a drop or two of an essential oil such as tea tree which is a powerful skin disinfectant that penetrates and helps heal infected areas very well. Add two tablespoons to your bath using the full flow of the hot tap and take a luxurious soak.

Birch bark, chamomile, clovers, comfrey root, marshmallow root, pansy, seaweed, white willow, and wintergreen, are all recommended as calming herbs. For psoriasis, take a bath with comfrey root mixed with white willow bark.

SOAK AND REJUVENATE!

For an antistress bath, try a combination of comfrey leaf, linden, patchouli, sandalwood, and savory in equal parts. Comfrey works against signs of aging, due to its high allantoin content. Allantoin promotes the growth of bone and cartilage and connective tissue, the latter being essential to healthy skin. Sandalwood improves skin tone, and savory is stimulating. This is balanced by linden, a natural antiseptic and relaxant, helping to produce a fortifying, antistress, and fragrant bath.

An herbal mixture recommended especially for long-term, repeated use to keep skin young-looking and firm uses 1 ounce each of aloe, comfrey root, lavender, lemon thyme, peppermint, rosemary, and fresh or dried roses. A little of this assortment works well on the body in various ways. The proven benefits of comfrey are supplemented by the cooling, healing astringency of aloe and roses. Lavender has a calming, antibacterial action, working well against acne and puffiness, and is reinforced by the roses, which also hydrate the skin. The menthol in peppermint is cooling and anesthetic as well as stimulating to the blood flow in skin. Thyme eases aches and pains and acts as a mild deodorant. Emerge from a soak in these herbs feeling fresh, clean and alive!

CHAPTER 11

Make Your Own Potpourri

Forget the disinfectants and air fresheners in a can! Go for natural, environmentally friendly fragrances instead. Simply hang up bunches of herbs chosen for their scent and their effects on mood. Try your hand, too, at combining dried herbs in potpourris, following recipes like the one below, or make up your own. Tip a little of each herb into a covered bowl to be exposed when occasional scent is desired, or into an open container for continuous fragrance. Stir the herbs and other ingredients together and sprinkle them with a few drops of an oil with a complementary odor.

Bring the scents of a flower garden indoors with five tablespoons of lavender flowers, three tablespoons each of carnations and scented rose petals, one and a half tablespoons each of chamomile flowers, heliotrope flowers, salt, and orris root powder. A little rose oil is a nice addition.

CHAPTER 12

Herbal Insect Repellents

The single most important reason that plants contain aromatic volatile oils is to repel insects! We can take advantage of this by using aromatic oils to repel pests, instead of the toxic petrochemical pesticides sold commercially. In fact, many of these substances can now be found at better plant and garden stores.

Pyrethrums, which come from plants in the chrysanthemum family, make potent insecticides as powder from the dried plants or spray infusions. Pyrethrum works by paralyzing insects and is so strong that prolonged contact can cause skin problems, so use it with care.

You can also make an infusion of 1 pound of elder leaves to 2 gallons of water as an effective aphid spray. And try a decoction of walnut leaves, six handfuls boiled for 20-30 minutes in one pint of water, to repel ants. Indoors, use southernwood, also known as garderobe (cothesguard), between sheets of tissue lain among clothes to keep moths away. Hanging bunches of herbs such as pennyroyal, rosemary, rue and tansy adds lovely scents to the summer air as they keep insects out of the house on summer evenings.

Venture out to flea-ridden grasses and the muggiest swamps wearing some of nature's own bug repellents! A short-term mosquito repellent is fresh elder. Simply rub the leaves on exposed parts, but be prepared to do this every twenty minutes. You can also make strong infusions of elder or chamomile to dab on frequently.

Citronella oil, made from the stone root plant, is a well known and longer-lasting bug deterrent. It also has a pleasant fragrance, and is much more effective and easier to apply than most store-bought insect repellents. Lavender oil is reputed to be similarly useful and has its own well-loved scent. Armed against bugs and perfumed as well—yet another typically effective, gentle and enjoyable result of using herbs!

Any of the plants with aromatic essential oils but especially pennyroyal, can also used as insect repellents.

CHAPTER 13

An Abbreviated Guide to Herbs and Illnesses

For	Use
Allergies	Ephedra, garlic
Arthritis	Cat's claw, arnica, feverfew, licorice, evening primrose, ginger
Cholesterol lowering	Garlic, ginger, hawthorn
Circulation	Ginkgo biloba, garlic, angelica, bilberry, calendula, ginger
Colds and flus	Echinacea, ephedra, garlic, goldenseal, elderberry
Cough	Licorice, ephedra, garlic, lavender
Depression, anxiety	Kava kava, St. John's wort
Digestion	Ginger, chamomile, the mints, fennel, angelica, licorice
Headache	Feverfew (migraine only), white willow bark, ginger, ginkgo, lavender, the mints
Heartburn	Licorice, the mints, fennel
Heart Strengthener	Hawthorn berries, garlic, dong quai

For	Use
Insomnia	Valerian, St. John's wort
Immune System Support	Echinacea, garlic, ginseng, angelica, cat's claw, goldenseal
Liver Support	Milk thistle
Lungs	Licorice, eucalyptus, garlic, ginseng, pennyroyal
Memory	Ginkgo biloba, kava
Menopause	Dong quai, vitex/chasteberry, angelica, licorice, ginseng
Pain	White willow bark, feverfew, arnica, licorice, aloe, calendula, cat's claw, echinacea, elderberry, kava, lavender
PMS	Vitex, dong quai, pennyroyal
Prostate	Saw palmetto
Sores, wounds, cuts and bruises, stings, bites and itches	Witch hazel, aloe vera, arnica, calendula
Urinary Tract	Uva ursi, saw palmetto
Vision	Bilberry

Sources and Resources

SOURCES

Barrie, N.D., "Effects of Garlic Oil on Platelet Aggregation, Serum Lipids and Blood Pressure in Humans," *Journal of Orthomolecular Medicine,* 1987, 2(1):15-21

Byrnes, P., "Wild Medicine," in *Wilderness,* The Wilderness Society, 1995, Vol.59, 210:28-33.

Farnsworth, N., et al., "Medicinal Plants in Therapy," *Bull World Health* Org., 1985, 63:965-981.

Fogarty, M., "Garlic's Potential Role in Reducing Heart Disease," *British Journal of Clinical Practice,* 1993, 47(2):64-65.

Hobbs, C., *The Echinacea Handbook,* Eclectic Medical Publications, Portland, OR, 1989.

Kowalchik, C., et al., *Rodale's Illustrated Encyclopedia of Herbs,* Rodale Press, Emmaus, Pennsylvania, 1987.

Lemley, B., Interview with Andrew Weil, *New Age Journal,* Dec. 1995:68.

Lust, J., *The Herb Book,* Bantam Books, New York, 1974.

Mabey, R., *The New Age Herbalist,* Collier Books, Macmillan Publishing Co., New York, 1988.

Macolo, N., et al., "Ethnopharmalogic Investigation of Ginger (Zingiber Officinale)," *J. Ethnopharmacol,* 1989, 27:129-140.

Mann, C., et al, "The Chemistry, Pharmacology, and Commercial Formulations of Chamomile," *Herbs Spices Med Plants,* 1985, 1:235-280.

Mindell, E., *Earl Mindell's Herb Bible,* Simon & Schuster/Fireside, New York, 1992.

Moore, Michael, *Medicinal Plants of the Mountain West,* Museum of New Mexico Press, Santa Fe, New Mexico, 1979.

Moore, Michael, *Medicinal Plants of the Pacific West,* Red Crane Books, Santa Fe, New Mexico, 1993.

Mowrey, Daniel B., Ph.D., *The Scientific Validation of Herbal Medicine*, Keats Publishing, New Canaan, CT, 1986.

Murray, M, *The Healing Power of Herbs*, Prima Publishing, California, 1995.

Rose, Jeanne, *Jeanne Rose's Herbal Body Book*, Perigree, Putnam Publishing, New York, 1976.

Tierra, Lesley, L.Ac., Herbalist, *The Herbs of Life: Health and Healing Using Western and Chinese Techniques*, The Crossing Press, Freedom, CA, 1992.

Vanderhoek, J., et al., "Inhibition of Fatty Acid Lipoxygenases by Onion and Garlic Oils. Evidence for the Mechanism by Which These Oils Inhibit Platelet Aggregation," *Bioch. Pharmacol.*, 1980, 29, 3:169-173.

Weiner, M., *Earth Medicine—Earth Food*, Fawcett Columbine, New York, 1980.

Werbach, Melvyn R. M.D., and Murray, Michael T, N.D., *Botanical Influences on Illness*, Third Line Press, Tarzana, California, 1994.

Willard, Terry, Ph.D., *The Wild Rose Scientific Herbal*, Wild Rose College of Natural Healing, Calgary, Alberta, 1991.

RESOURCES

For more information on herbal medicines contact the following organizations:

The American Botanical Council
P.O. Box 201660
Austin, TX 78720
(512) 331-8868

The Herb Research Foundation
1007 Pearl Street, Ste. 200
Boulder, CO 80302
(303) 449-2265

An **excellent guide to alternative medicine health care professionals** is *The Alternative Medicine Yellow Pages*, $12.95. It is also available in many bookstores. It is published by:

   Future Medicine Publishing
   98 Main Street, Ste. 209
   Tiburon, CA 94920

For referrals to naturopathic physicians write or call:
   American Association of Naturopathic Physicians
   P.O. Box 20386
   Seattle, WA 98102
   (206) 323-7610

For referrals to Chinese Medicine Doctors, contact:
   American Association of Acupuncture and
   Oriental Medicine
   4101 Lake Boone Trail, Ste. 201
   Raleigh, NC 27607
   (919) 787-5181

Index

Dr. Earl Mindell's

What You Should Know About...
series
in print or forthcoming